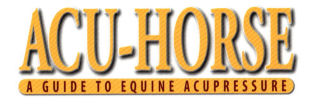

Nancy Zidonis
Amy Snow

Foreword by
Madalyn Ward, DVM

Tallgrass Publishers, LLC

Castle Pines, CO

Tallgrass Publishers, LLC.
Castle Pines, Colorado
www.tallgasspublishers.com
tallgrass@animalacupressure.com

Copyright ©2013 Tallgrass Publishers, LLC. All rights reserved. Printed in the United States of America. No part of this book may be reproduced or transmitted in any form or by any means, electronic or mechanical, including photocopying, recording, internet, or by any information storage and retrieval system without written permission from the publisher.

ISBN 978-1-936796-04-5
    1. Horses 2. Equine Health 3. Complementary Veterinary Medicine
    4. Animal Acupressure 5. Equine Health 6. Equine Acupressure
    7. Equine Massage Therapy 8. Alternative Animal Healthcare
    9. Traditional Chinese Medicine

FIRST EDITION

Library of Congress Cataloging-in-Publication Data

Book & Cover Design: Grant Dunmire, Attention Media Group,
    Las Vegas, Nevada
Cover & Back Cover Photographs: John Wiet Photography,
    www.johnwiet.com

Technical Editing: KimBauer, Lead Instructor,
    Tallgrass Animal Acupressure Institute
Illustrations: Carla Stroh, Lusk, Wyoming
Anatomical Drawings: Janet Goldman-Merrill, San Pedro, California

Note: This book is intended as an informational guide. The approaches and techniques described herein are meant to complement and not be a substitute for professional veterinary care. They should not be used to treat any ailment, injury, or sudden behavior change without prior consultation with a qualified healthcare practitioner. It is recommended that horses receive regular visits with a holistic veterinarian.

Foreword

What a privilege to be asked to write the foreword for *ACU-HORSE: A Guide to Equine Acupressure*. Having written several holistic horse care books myself, I understand the time, energy, and labor of love required to produce a high-quality product. Authors Amy Snow and Nancy Zidonis have put together a book that's not only well written but also extremely valuable as a handbook to help owners care for their horses.

My journey into holistic medicine has been a long process. Upon graduating from Texas A&M veterinary school in 1980, I was sure that my education had prepared me perfectly to heal horses and improve their lives. However, after 10 years of conventional practice, I was sorely disappointed. I spent most of my time treating acute and chronic conditions and realized I had little to offer clients to *prevent* illness in their horses. Then in 1993, I was introduced to acupressure for horses and my world opened up to true holistic healing.

Holistic medicine offered new ways for me to look at patterns of disease and health. Wanting to heal on a deep level, I discovered the need for balance in a horse's internal systems to be more important than external symptoms. Horses are extremely sensitive to shifts in their energetic patterns, which makes them excellent candidates for acupressure.

One of the beautiful things about acupressure is that while correct application will yield better results than incorrect application, doing it wrong can't hurt the horse. Acupressure involves no pain, and horses learn to love the sensations they experience. It's not uncommon for a horse to indicate with its nose the points it wants the acupuncturist to work on. By the same token, if a horse doesn't enjoy stimulation of a point, it may move away or show annoyance. What a wonderful way to build a relationship of trust with a horse.

I always have *ACU-HORSE: A Guide to Equine Acupressure* within reach when I work on horses. The descriptions of the acupressure points enhance understanding of Traditional Chinese Medicine principles. In addition, the points selected for different conditions provide a blueprint for bringing the horse back into a healthy state based on foundational healing, not just removal of symptoms.

Whether the intention is to treat an imbalance or solely to make a routine grooming session more beneficial, acupressure can benefit any horse care program.

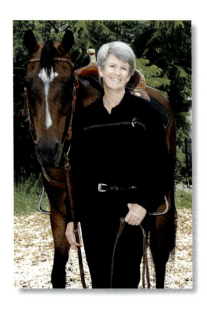

— **Madalyn Ward, DVM**

Author of: *Holistic Horsekeeping*
Horse Harmony
Horse Harmony Feeding Guide
www.holistichorsekeeping.com

Contents

Foreword – Madalyn Ward, DVM — iii

Introduction – Ancient Healing and Equine Health — vii

Chapter One – THE EVOLUTION AND NATURE OF THE HORSE — 1

Chapter Two – EQUINE ACUPRESSURE AND TRADITIONAL CHINESE MEDICINE — 9
   Barefoot Doctors
   Horses, You, and TCM

Reference: CUN MEASUREMENT — 12

Chapter Three - Key Concepts of Traditional Chinese Medicine — 13
   Universal Law
   Law of Integrity

Chapter Four – THEORY OF CHI — 17
   Five Functions of Chi   Harmonious Flow of Chi
   Major Types of Chi

Chapter Five – THEORY OF YIN - YANG — 23
   Nature of Yin and Yang   Four Patterns of Disharmony
   Pattern of Harmony

Chapter Six – Five-Element Theory — 33
   Balance and the Five Elements   Five Element Theory Cycles
   Correspondences of the Elements   Differentiating Patterns

Chapter Seven – ZANG-FU AND MERIDIAN THEORY — 43
   Zang-fu Theory   Meridians
   Organ Systems

Chapter Eight – 12 MAJOR MERIDIANS AND 2 EXTRAORDINARY VESSELS — 51
   Meridians and Acupressure   Stomach - Spleen
   Zang-Fu Organ System Functions   Heart - Small Intestine
   Indicators and Assessment   Bladder - Kidney
   Acupoint Selection   Pericardium - Triple Heater
   Lung - Large Intestine   Gall Bladder - Liver
                                 Conception - Governing Vessel

Chapter Nine – ASSESSING YOUR HORSE — 101
   Assessment process - The Four Examinations
   Association and Alarm Points
   Quick Review of the Assessment Process
   Interpretation for Assessment Purposes

Chapter Ten – EQUINE ACUPRESSURE SESSION PROTOCOL   117
    Acupressure Protocol   Acupoint Selection
    Association Points, Back *Shu* Points   Muddy Water
    Alarm Points, Front *Mu* Points   Closing
                                                         Post-Session

Chapter Eleven – EQUINE SPECIFIC CONDITIONS   139
    Local and Distal Acupoints
    Equine Aging Issues
        General Aging Issues
    Osteoarthritis
        Joints Exhibit Heat   Worse With Cold Weather
        Migrating Pain   Worse With Wet Weather

    Behavior Issues
        Cribbing   Focus On Training
        Fear   Grief
                                        Nervousness / Anxiety

    Gastrointestinal Issues
        Flatulent Colic   Prevention of Colic
        Impaction Colic   Improve Digestion
                                  Diarrhea / Constipation

    General Conditions
        Immune System Issues   Edema
        Immune System Strengthening   Hoof Problems / Founder

    Musculoskeletal Issues
        Cervical / Neck Issues   Post-Performance
        Hock Issues   Shoulder Soreness
        Lower Back Soreness   Stifle Issues
        Pre-Performance   Tying-Up

    Equine Reproduction
        Fertility Issues   Insufficient Lactation

    Respiratory Conditions
        General Lung Support   Heaves

    Sensory Issue
        Visual Acuity   Conjunctivitis

    Trauma
        Anhidrosis   Heatstroke
        Shock

Glossary   191

Bibliography   208

Index   209

Photographic Credits   213

Author Profiles   215

Introduction

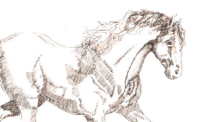

ANCIENT HEALING AND EQUINE HEALTH

Since the beginning of human history, the horse has been our constant companion in farming, war, travel, and sport. These powerful animals have played an important role in human survival worldwide. Because of the horse's athleticism, intelligence, and adaptability, humans have forged a bond between our two species that will never be broken.

When we domesticated the horse, we also took on the responsibility of caring for horses. We realized if we were going to rely on the horse's strength for food production, travel, military purposes, and communication across distances, then we'd best take good care of this living, breathing resource.

The ancient Chinese were well aware of their dependence on horses and the need for their horses to be healthy. Acupressure-massage has been used with both humans and domesticated animals for thousands of years in the vast countryside of China. Equine acupressure-massage charts that document the use of these ancient healing techniques still exist. What started as tribal healing evolved over thousands of years into a more pervasive and codified science. Fortunately, Traditional Chinese Medicine (TCM) has been passed down from generation to generation.

Modern medicine has finally "caught up to" traditional medicine. Current conventional veterinary medicine has also begun to see the value of integrating modern technology with a form of medicine that has thousands of years of clinical observation to support it. Both approaches to medicine have their place in caring for ourselves and our horses. By combining the strengths of each form of medicine, we can reap the benefit of health and well-being.

Acupressure-massage, called *Tui-Na* in Chinese, is noninvasive, always available, deceptively gentle, yet profoundly powerful. Horses have proven to be excellent candidates for the healing nature of acupressure because they're highly attuned to their internal energetics and sensitive to external, physical stimuli. Just think of how the horse wards off a fly even before it lands on him. Also, when horses stampede, they rarely, if ever, bump into each other.

Acupressure offers you a way to actively participate in your horse's health. It gives you a means of building a close partnership with your horse and his well-being, and contributes to years of quality performance and mutual enjoyment.

Acupressure has consistently been proven to:
- strengthen muscles, tendons, joints, and bones
- enhance mental clarity and calm required for focus
- release natural cortisone to reduce swelling and inflammation
- increase lubrication of the joints for better movement
- release endorphins to increase energy and relieve pain
- resolve injuries more quickly by increasing blood supply
- balance energy to optimize the body's ability to perform.

In Chapter One of *ACU-HORSE: A Guide to Equine Acupressure*, we delve into the TCM theories and concepts underlying acupressure. Subsequent chapters take you step by step through application of this rich traditional medicine. Once you have a firm grasp of these ancient Chinese ideas and practice their application, you'll gain insight into your horse's health and be able to help him feel and perform at his best.

Please note that acupressure isn't a substitute for veterinary medical care. Rather, it serves to complement medical services. Therefore, when your horse is ill or injured, seek appropriate medical attention from a qualified veterinary practitioner.

Horses are particularly receptive and responsive to acupressure. They want and need to bond with their human. With acupressure, you can provide them with this rich, shared experience, both for their health and this close connection.

ACU-HORSE provides a key that will help you unlock your healing ability as well as assist your horse in fulfilling his promise.

"The horse, with beauty unsurpassed, strength immeasurable and grace unlike any other, still remains humble enough to carry a man upon his back."

— Amber Senti

Chapter One

The Evolution and Nature of the Horse

If it weren't for a few strategic evolutionary advantages, we wouldn't be sharing our hearts and lives with horses at all. The evolution of the equid has been serious business. It's taken 55 million years to arrive at the horse we know and love today.

Evolutionary History

Over thousands of years, horses evolved from small, compact animals to animals with large bodies and long legs, which gave them the advantage of speed. When their habitat of tropical and dense forests disappeared and turned to grass lands, their loss of food sources could have wiped them out—but it didn't. Even with their large bodies, they adapted to eating low-nutrient forage. The teeth and internal digestive system of these grazers evolved in response to the environmental change.

The expansion of the equid's neocortex about 55 million years ago resulted in a huge evolutionary advantage. Because the neocortex of the brain is responsible for learning, memory, and managing sensory input, this attribute alone could have made the difference between survival and extinction.

As prey animals and grassland grazers, horses had a lot of adapting to do. The spring action of their legs helped propel them to safety. To increase speed and outrun predators, the single hoof won out over toes. Having a long head with eyes quite a bit above the ground helped horses remain watchful while they grazed. Even their digestive system gave them the advantage of being able to eat and run in a flash.

A distinctly opportune event for the modern horse occurred about 6,000 years ago. The Eurasian steppe dwellers realized the horse—the power of the beast—could be a tremendous resource. Until then, they had hunted wild horses for meat, which brought them to the brink of extinction. When humans recognized they could use horses for other purposes, the horse was saved by domestication, benefiting all concerned.

How did this come about? Horses began pilfering from the cultivated fields surrounding human settlements, and being closer to human habitat, they were better protected from predators. Over time, the more curious, dependent, and submissive horses blended with human civilization. When this happened, the modern horse and human history began to develop in tandem.

This mutual compatibility led to humans breeding horses, which gave the domestication of the horse a significant boost. All the horses' evolutionary strategies made them perfect candidates for survival among humans. Their pliant nature, speed, power, size, and intelligence gave them the edge over many other animals lost to extinction.

It's the domesticated horse's amazing adaptability that affords it a place in our world today. Horses can eat a variety of foods; they can sustain their bodies on minimal nutrient forage. They're relatively docile animals that can be trained for a wide variety of human-related activities, from pulling plows and carriages to carrying people on their backs in warfare and sport.

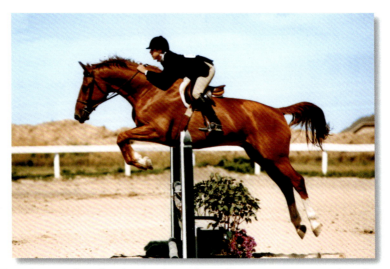

Historians and archeologists have long been piecing together facts and assumptions concerning the horse's role in the growth of civilization. Many a legend and excavation have given us a glimpse of what could have happened. We know for sure, however, that horses have been at our side for thousands of years and have served us well, no matter what we've demanded of them.

Anatomical Marvels

With all the adaptations the horse has had to make physically, the modern horse's large, muscular body is truly an anatomical marvel. What an astounding job horses have done surviving, evolving, and reproducing.

Their long necks and sensitive, prehensile lips are perfect for grazing on forage. The rough, cellulose material is ground into mash by their powerful jaws and the transverse shearing action of their teeth to form a saliva-infused bolus that can travel up through the esophagus and down into the stomach.

For the size of the animal, the equine stomach is relatively small. Enzymes act upon the cellulose material in the stomach and some nutrients are extracted. Luckily, and sometimes not so luckily, the horse has a fairly large, u-shaped cecum where much of the fermentation process occurs to create bio-absorbable nutrients. Because material enters at the top of the cecum and the remaining material also has to exit at the top of the cecum, this can present a problem if the horse is not able to drink a sufficient amount of water.

From the cecum, what's left of the fluid and material passes into the large colon, where microbial digestion continues for anywhere from 48 to 65 hours. And finally, the indigestible waste passes into the small colon. Fluids are extracted from the waste, forming fecal balls that pass from the rectum.

In the wild, horses traverse 20 to 40 miles in a day to meet their needs for forage and water. This consistent movement greatly enhances the motility of their digestive system. Our domesticated horses, on the other hand, are often limited in the amount of exercise and choice of feed they have, which contributes to digestive issues.

Being a prey animal created a lot of opportunity for physical adaptation for horses. Because they needed to keep a watchful eye for predators, horses can see almost 360 degrees. Their vigilance was enhanced by the fact that they needed only two or so hours of deep sleep in 24 hours. In addition, the horse's passive stay apparatus ("locking" or stabilizing of the fore and hind limb joints) gives him the ability to rest and sleep lightly while standing—another exceptional protective adaptation.

The horse's entire body is an amazing mechanical feat of nature. His large, muscular body is carried on thin legs below the carpus and stifle.

This design means the horse can run at high speeds because the lower portions of his legs have no bulky muscles to slow him down.

At a full gallop, the horse's diaphragm acts like a bellows moving forward and backward, forcing air in and out of his lungs with each stride. This saves muscle power expended in leg movement. Think how efficient it is for an animal that depends on flight rather than fight for his existence.

A lot of the horse's brain power is devoted to his body. The horse's brain is in charge of every movement he makes. To survive, he needs to know where his feet are at all times. There's a good reason why a foal has to get up on her feet and be able to get going with the herd within two hours of being born. Horses tend to have only one offspring a year, and if the foals weren't ready to move quickly right away, they wouldn't be around very long due to predators. Hence, motor skills and muscle development are present at birth.

Horses are curious, have long memories, can learn, and can generalize information. The crack of a whip carries a clear association for any horse that's experienced a whip connecting with his body. If a branch of a tree breaks and makes a similar cracking sound, that horse will have the same response as he did to the whip cracking. Responding and coming to the sound of grain in a bucket is another stimulus-response learned behavior.

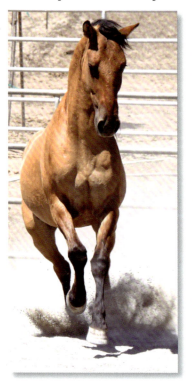

Horses have adapted to carrying us on their backs and pulling us along in wagons. They've learned to walk, trot, and canter on demand, changing their natural conformation and gait to please our notion of how a horse should look when he moves. To fulfill our desire, horses will even jump over obstacles they can't see or judge ahead of time. These magnificent animals have learned how to adapt to human expectations as part of their continuing survival strategy.

The Horse's Social Structure

The equine social herd structure is perfect for grassland animals as well as for domesticated animals. The herd provides protection in the open spaces, the ability to find resources, and a defined source for reproduction. Each stallion has his harem of mares, which varies in number depending on the ages of offspring and less-dominant males staying with the herd.

The hierarchical herd structure is based on dominance. The dominant mare is the leader. She determines where the herd will go to find food and water. The stallion is the protector of the herd and will follow the herd, watching for any threat and warding off any intruders. For the most part, this structure creates stability and peace within the herd.

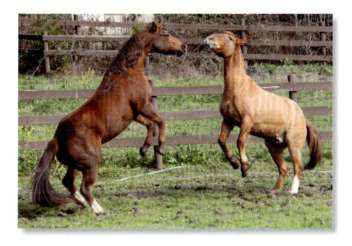

To maintain the health and vigor of any social or biological system, challenges need to be prevalent. A young stallion will challenge an old stallion. A younger mare will take on an older mare. They will compete for resources, and the strongest animal will win the dominant position within the herd. Once the pecking order is established, the herd returns to calm, cooperative herd behavior.

The herd's survival depends on its cohesiveness. This means the horses usually don't fight to the death or display crippling aggression. Their challenges are often more show and less real striking and biting. The more submissive animal is apt to back down after a bit of posturing. Horses know the body language of ear-pinning, neck-extending, and other aggressive behaviors. These bluffs serve to avoid serious aggression. That's not to say there can't be a nasty clash in which a horse is badly hurt, but it's rare.

Young stallions will band together and leave in search of their own harems rather than battle for dominance within their original herd. Mares tend to bond with each other and form friendships for mutual grooming, protecting the young, managing access to food and water, and maintaining stability. Thus the herd is a cohesive, hierarchical social structure that provides each member the best chance for survival.

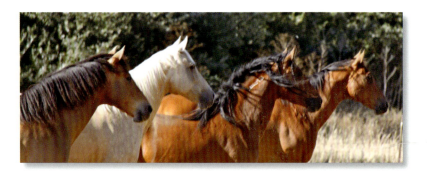

Domestication of Horses

Why did wild horses become domesticated? Was it simply their better chance of survival on the fringes of human habitation that eventually brought them under our dominance? Initially, that had a lot to do with it, but another twist of evolution seems to have played a big part in domestication.

Once horses came closer to humans, they became more dependent on us for food. The closer they came, the more we found ways to dominate them, including controlling their breeding. Selective breeding then led to a less independent horse. Over thousands of years, horses increasingly exhibited youthful traits into adulthood, a phenomenon called neoteny. Equine neoteny behavior traits include curiosity, submissiveness, playfulness, adaptability, and a willingness to be cared for. Add neoteny to the horse's capacity to bond and equine social structure, and the result is the domesticated horse.

Due to their hierarchical social structure, horses have accepted our dominance, and we've used them for entertainment, military, and economic gain for centuries. Of late, however, human consciousness has shifted. Our humanity is finally catching up with us, and we're seeing horses as beings with hearts and minds, which makes them our companions. In fact, how we treat our horses is a measure of our humanity.

Yes, horses have adapted to domestication—yet they have the same flesh, bones, and internal workings as the wild horses still roaming the hidden ranges. We have to consider the stress we cause by imposing our need for convenience on them. After all, we keep them in small spaces, and that alone can bring about self-destructive, obsessive-compulsive equine behavior. Can you imagine what a horse that's self-destructive must be feeling?

To minimize the stress and add to our relationship with our horses, we can provide as natural an environment as possible, pay attention to their nutrient requirements, and adhere to positive training techniques. Learning and including equine acupressure in caring for our horses creates a special bond they will treasure as much as we do.

> **"The almost magical cooperation of horse and rider is testimony both to the inventiveness of man and to the remarkable learning ability and physical prowess of the horse."**
> — Stephen Budiansky,
> *The Nature of Horses*

Key Traditional Chinese Medicine Concepts & Theories

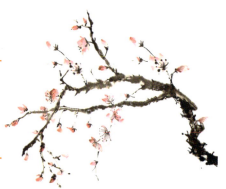

Universal Law of Nature	The human or horse body is an integral part of nature.
Law of Integrity	When an imbalance occurs internally, it will manifest externally.
Chi	Life-promoting force intrinsic to all living beings.
Yin/Yang	The two opposite yet complementary and interdependent aspects of chi that are in constant dynamic balance.
Zang-Fu Organs	Internal organ systems.
Meridians	The energetic channels or pathways that are extensions of the internal organs along which chi and blood flow to nourish the body.
Five-Element or Five Phases of Transformation	A conceptual model representing the natural phases of life cycle and seasonal transformation

Chapter Two

EQUINE ACUPRESSURE AND TRADITIONAL CHINESE MEDICINE

The ancient Chinese knew animals and humans lived by the same laws of the natural world. Seasonal shifts affect all of us in similar ways. In the spring, we feel more energetic than we did in the frigid winter. In summer when the earth is verdant green, horses graze on rich grasses, rest during the midday heat, graze, and play in the cool mornings and evenings. We enjoy all the activity we can in the long summer days. Autumn is the time when animals and humans reap and prepare for winter.

The Chinese paid close attention to the natural cycles of days, seasons, and life. They saw that when we all live in harmony with the natural climatic cycles, people and animals live longer, healthier lives. In winter, for instance, it's best to retain internal body heat, eat warming foods, focus internally, and not expend a lot of energy. Spring is a time to be more active, eat fresh foods, and build strength to get ready for summer's even higher activity level.

Because it's based on the tenets of the natural world, Chinese medicine requires a different mindset than western medicine—a more poetic way of thinking. The ancient Chinese used the world they knew to describe health issues. For instance, "damp cold" refers to an edema, which is encapsulated fluid that has no heat or energy moving or warming it. Another example is what we call heatstroke and Chinese medicine calls summer heat, indicating extremely dangerous heat.

The ancient Chinese relied on their knowledge of how beings function within their environment day to day, season to season, and in each phase of life. How well is this animal or human functioning within his environment? That's the question they asked. Is this horse coping well in the spring when the winds are blowing? Are his tendons and ligaments flexible enough for increased spring training? How is this horse dealing with the sudden cold spells in the autumn? Does this animal have respiratory issues during the fall as temperatures cool down?

Horses, You, and TCM

Acupressure connects you and your horse to thousands of years of natural healing. Though Chinese medicine can seem complex, you can learn the underlying concepts and theories and be able to work with your own horses. All horses want to feel good and when they do, they show it. Working with your horse is gratifying because you're contributing to his well-being.

Let's begin by building a foundation consisting of Traditional Chinese Medicine theories and concepts. These ideas distinguish Chinese medicine from all other forms of medicine. The following chapters delve into these key concepts and theories in detail, but below is a quick overview.

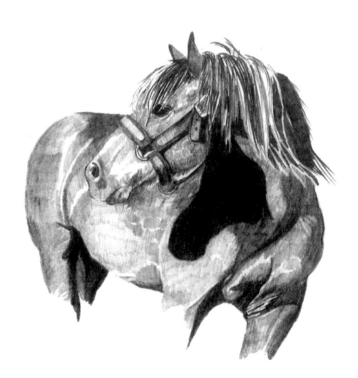

In Traditional Chinese Medicine (TCM), we look at each horse in his entirety within his environment and recognize that each horse is unique. Thus, our approach to managing his health and happiness is specific to him. Emotions are as important as the physical being because they have an equally strong impact on the animal's wellness. The horse's mind-body-spirit is a unique and integrated whole.

When a horse becomes ill, it means he's not able to cope within his environment. From a TCM perspective, most illness is considered a breakdown of the immune system in some manner. When the body's natural defenses aren't strong, external climatic pathogens such as wind, cold, and heat can "invade" the body and illness can occur. In addition, internal stresses such as extreme anger or excessive grieving can injure the immune system and lead to illness.

Chinese medicine—both ancient and the way it's practiced today—promotes supporting the immune system by living a natural, balanced lifestyle. Horses have the same needs we do: proper food, exercise, rest, play, social interaction, caring, and touch. These basic needs can be further supported by acupressure-massage.

Barefoot Doctors

The practice of TCM is the practice of preventive care. Hundreds of years ago, "barefoot doctors" would go from village to village, and they'd receive housing, food, and payment only when the community was healthy. The reasoning was simple: When the community was not well (including horses, livestock, and other animals in the community), it meant the barefoot doctor was not doing a good job, so why should the community reward him?

When the community was well, it lavished the doctor with riches, food, and elegant accommodations. The Chinese realized it's smarter to sustain good health rather than wait until the immune system is weak and the person or animal falls prey to illness. Hence, Chinese medicine has always focused on health rather than illness. Its purpose is to help the body adapt to constant environmental and internal changes.

ACU-HORSE: A Guide To Equine Acupressure

Reference: Cun Measurement

In Chinese medicine, cun measurement is used to locate acupoints. Cun, pronounced "tsun," means "little measurement." A cun measurement is relative and proportional to the conformation of each individual horse. A cun measurement identifies the distance from one anatomical landmark to another or one acupoint to another. Because horses vary in size and conformation, the length of a cun on a Thoroughbred is going to be larger than on a Shetland pony. The cun provides a more accurate method of measurement than inches or centimeters because it is specific to a particular horse's body.

There are a number of methods of determining the length of a cun. For an average size horse, you can use the distance from the center of the elbow to the center of the horse's carpus (wrist) to determine a cun. There are 12 cun between the horse's elbow and carpus. An easy way to find the cun is to divide the space between the elbow and carpus in half. Then divide the space from the middle of the leg to the carpus in half again. The distance between that lower-quarter of the leg above the carpus is automatically three (3) cun. You can continue to break it down to arrive at one (1) cun.

Another example in how to determine a cun measurement for a horse is to measure the distance from the shoulder joint to the elbow crease on the foreleg. Simply divide that distance into three equal portions and you will be able to measure 3 cun. Compare this to the finger-width of your hand to be able to use this measurement in locating acupoints. If you know 3 cun and the location calls for 1 cun, divide the distance by 3 and you will know how to measure 1 cun.

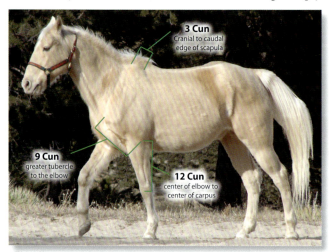

This diagram provides a number of alternative methods of arriving at a cun measurement for each individual horse.

Chapter Three

KEY CONCEPTS OF TRADITIONAL CHINESE MEDICINE

Chinese medicine began as folk medicine practiced in the small villages throughout the vast countryside of China thousands of years ago. It's believed that the first known text, *The Classic of Internal Medicine*, or *Neijing Suwen*, was written by Huang Di, known as the Yellow Emperor, during the Warring States period (475–221 BCE).

Legend holds that Huang Di and his trusted doctor friend Qi Bo discussed the conceptual basis of TCM in two texts, *Miraculous Pivot* and *Plain Questions*. These texts summarize the collected medical knowledge for the prevention and treatment of disease.

In his recent translation of *The Essential Text of Chinese Health and Healing: The Yellow Emperor's Classic of Medicine*, Maoshing Ni, Ph.D. sums up the core sense of Chinese medicine in the Preface:

> The Neijing offers much practical advice on how to maintain balance by revealing the inner workings of the universal law. The environment, the way of life, and the spirit all contribute to the quality of human existence. The essence of the Neijing can be summed up in the following passage: "Health and well-being can be achieved only by remaining centered, guarding against squandering of energy, promoting the constant flow of qi and blood, maintaining a harmonious balance of yin and yang, adapting to the changing seasons and yearly macrocosmic influences, and nourishing one's self preventively. This is the way to a long and happy life."

The *Neijing* became the foundation for TCM by describing the origin of disease and defining the principles for identifying and treating diseases.

During ancient times, it must have taken years for information to travel from one part of China to another. Even though communication was difficult, the theories and even the energetics of specific acupressure points (also called acupoints) were, and are, much the same today as they were centuries ago. Isn't it amazing to think of how this body of knowledge has arrived at our modern doorstep with such cohesive and coherent content?

From antiquity to present, Chinese medicine has evolved and proven to be a rich resource for natural healing. The Chinese have contributed an astounding amount of knowledge to medicine. At least six thousand books have been written about TCM theory and technique. Currently, we're experiencing a shift back to traditional forms of medicine for both humans and horses because these forms bring the body back to a healthy balance.

TCM consists of theories, with two essential concepts inherent in the theories. The first is the Universal Law of Nature and the second is the Law of Integrity.

Universal Law of Nature

The first major concept underlying Traditional Chinese Medicine is the idea that humans and animals are an integral part of nature. We're all subject to elements and forces of our natural environment. As part of the natural world, we must live in harmony with nature. The living body-mind-spirit must be both strong and flexible enough to adapt to environmental change.

For our body to remain healthy and balanced in the winter, we need to stay warm, not over-exercise, eat warming foods, be internally focused, and sleep when it's dark to adapt to the cold environment. In the summer, we can be more active, eat cooling foods, be more social, get less sleep, and enjoy the warmth of the season. Likewise, we can support our horse's natural ability to shift and adapt when the climate dictates.

> ... "It is a general law that generation occurs in spring, growth in summer, gathering in autumn, and storage in winter—we must act accordingly."
>
> — Huang Di and Qi Bo, Treatise on the Variations of Chi During the Day, *Miraculous Pivot*

When left to their own ways of living in the wild, horses follow the Universal Law of Nature for their survival. They have an inner knowing of how to balance their lifestyles during the ever-changing seasons and cycles of life. Wild horses know which grasses to eat throughout the year, and they're completely capable of adapting their expenditure of physical energy to the climate. Plus, horses live within the social network of their herd for protection and reproduction.

Law of Integrity

The Law of Integrity is the notion that the body is an integrated system. That is, the body is a single entity in which all of the parts must function optimally for the animal to be balanced and healthy. If there's an imbalance—for example, an internal organ is not able to function properly—the imbalance will be evident on the external, superficial part of the body.

For instance, when the liver isn't healthy, the whites of the eyes turn yellow, which is the external manifestation of liver disease. Another example is when a horse has a drippy nose and his breathing sounds congested. These are the outward manifestations indicating a respiratory imbalance. The horse is showing signs that his lungs aren't functioning optimally.

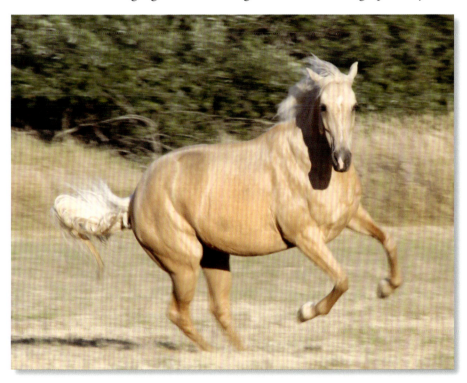

The Law of Integrity is the basis of the holistic approach to medicine. What's occurring internally will manifest externally. We know a healthy horse when we see one: his eyes are bright and alert, his muscles articulate with every step, his coat is sleek and shiny, and his hooves are strong, not chipped or cracked. Every movement emanates his joy in being alive. This horse is perfectly adapted to his environment with all his internal organs functioning properly; he's one whole, vital animal.

The Universal Law of Nature and the Law of Integrity are the significant underpinnings for the TCM theories. It's important for you to have a sense of how the Chinese viewed the living body in relation to its place in the world and within itself. These two ideas are pervasive throughout Chinese medicine.

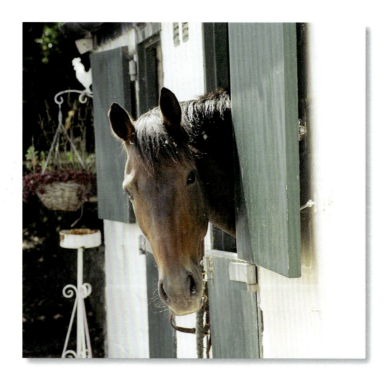

Chapter Four

THEORY OF CHI

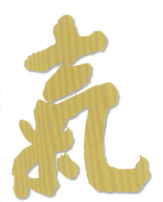

In Taoist philosophy, all that exists in the universe was created by invisible *chi*. Chi is often described as the life-promoting force that flows throughout the body. Its presence or absence means the difference between being alive or dead. Chi enlivens the human or horse body. All living things embody chi.

The ancient Chinese were most interested in the spark of life. They wanted to understand how this magical, energetic force functioned to animate the body. Chi has to exist for life to exist because when it's gone, the body is dead and, in time, disintegrates into dust.

In terms of Chinese medicine, chi is responsible for all of the body's vital functions. It flows along invisible yet very real pathways or channels throughout the body to nourish the internal organs, all bodily tissues, and consciousness.

The Five Functions of Chi

How does chi function to keep the body alive? Chi must perform five functions to support balanced health:

1. **Promoting** – Chi is responsible for all of the physiological activities of the internal organ systems and production of vital substances, including blood circulation and distribution of body fluids.

2. **Warming** – Chi must maintain the temperature of the body; chi is the warmth of the body.

3. **Defending** (*Wei Chi / Zheng Chi*) – Chi defends the exterior of the body so that no external pathogens such as heat, wind, dry, wet, or cold can invade and disrupt the flow of chi. Chi defends the body from internal stress such as the volatility of emotions.

4. **Controlling** – Chi controls and regulates the functioning of the body's substances. To create balance within the body, there must also be control. For instance, if chi were not controlling urination, the animal would experience incontinence.

5. **Activating** (*Chi Hua*) – Chi activates all bodily processes. Chi is responsible for the transformation of essential substances within the organs. Examples include when the activity of digestion transforms food into bio-absorbable nutrients and when body fluids are transformed into blood.

These functions are actually inseparable. As the "root" of living activity in the body, all of these functions must act in unison and combine to create balance necessary to sustain life. To further illustrate how important the notion of chi is to Traditional Chinese Medicine, scholars went on to identify many different types of chi required to support life.

Major Types of Chi

The purpose in identifying different types of chi is to be able to distinguish exactly which type of chi is not functioning well when there are indicators the horse is experiencing some kind of dysfunction. When a horse shows signs of an allergic reaction, we know that his immune system is not as strong as it should be.

For instance, allergies are seen as an immune system breakdown because the body isn't able to defend itself from an environmental allergen. Identifying and knowing the issue gives us the opportunity to strengthen the horse's immune system so he can cope with allergens present in the environment.

The first type of chi is Source chi because its presence indicates that life has begun for the animal.

Source Chi, *Yuan Chi.* This is the original essence chi (*Jing Chi*) that the horse inherits from his dam and sire. If the dam and sire are thoroughbreds, the offspring will be a thoroughbred. Source chi is the basic conformation of the animal; the essence of the body. According to TCM, the foal arrives on earth with a certain amount of Source chi, also called Prenatal chi, Congenital chi, or Heavenly chi, which dissipates throughout the horse's life. In other words, at birth, the horse has as much original essence chi as he will ever have. It serves to help him grow to maturity and reproduce. The Original chi diminishes throughout the horse's life until it can no longer sustain him and death ensues.

Source chi determines the conformation and general health of the horse. When the dam, for instance, has too many foals in succession and her body has become depleted, the odds are high of having a weak, unhealthy foal. The dam doesn't have enough Source chi left to support healthy offspring.

In general, the original Source chi, which is stored in the Kidney, is responsible for the growth, development, reproduction, and life-long functioning of the entire body.

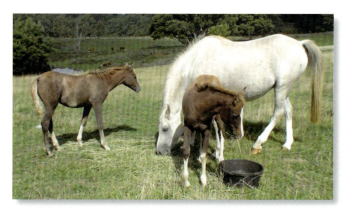

Pectoral Chi, *Zong Chi.* This form of chi is also called Chest chi and Gathering chi. It's created by inhaling air, which is then transformed into usable oxygen (*Qing Chi*) in the Lung. Pectoral chi is considered an Acquired chi or Post Heavenly chi because it's created after birth. Pectoral chi is chi acquired to sustain life. If the horse's lungs are not able to transform oxygen into pectoral chi, the horse will not survive.

Nutrient Chi, *Ying Chi.* This is another form of Acquired chi. Nutrient chi is derived from the forage the horse eats. The forage is broken down into absorbable nutrients by the Spleen, according to TCM, while held in the stomach. Once the fermentation process, or "rotting and ripening" process, is complete, the highly refined Nutrient chi ascends to combine with Pectoral chi and is transformed into Protective chi, *Wei Chi*, and True Chi *(Zhen Chi)* which is sent to the heart to become nutrient-rich blood.

Nutrient chi and Pectoral chi are two forms of Acquired chi necessary for the horse to have a healthy, long life. Even though the horse consumes relatively low-nutrient grasses, as long as the grass has the right balance of nutrients, his body can utilize it effectively. Having clean air to breathe is important for overall health. The quality of these two forms of Acquired chi support Source chi, making it possible for the horse to live as long as possible.

> "The point where pathogenic factors invade the body is bound to be a place where chi is deficient."
>
> — Treatise on Fevers from *Plain Questions* by Huang Di & Qi Bo

Immune System Chi, ***Wei Chi*** **and** ***Zheng Chi.*** The horse's immune system must be strong to ward off external pathogens (*Xie Chi*) and internal stress. *Wei Chi* protects the more superficial portions of the body from the invasion of external pathogens. When there's a cold wind blowing, it's the *Wei Chi* that defends the horse. The Lung is responsible for sending this "protective" or "defensive" chi to the surface of the body, which includes the skin and muscles.

Zheng Chi is the body's total immune system. It's based on the proper functioning of the internal organ systems along with the strength of the *Wei Chi*. *Zheng Chi* is the body's ability to resist internal or external pathogens. The horse's body will not fall prey to illness when *Zheng Chi* is strong.

Harmonious Flow of Chi

The concept of chi distinguishes Chinese medicine from all other types of medicine. Many more different types of chi have been identified than we describe in this book. The TCM practitioner is interested in figuring out how chi is performing to support vitality and health. By isolating and naming different functions of chi, the practitioner can figure out what's not working well.

For example, say a horse is having respiratory issues in autumn when the winds are cold. The practitioner will know the protective chi, *Wei Chi,* isn't strong. The Lung is responsible for the distribution of Protective chi and is not doing its job well enough to keep the horse healthy. The practitioner will use acupoints known to support the health of the Lung organ system.

Another example is when a horse's muscles aren't as strong or full as they were a month or so ago, even though his exercise level hasn't changed. This can mean the muscle tissue isn't absorbing enough nourishment. When Nutrient chi is deficient, the practitioner knows to check to see if the Spleen is functioning as well as it should to supply refined, absorbable nutrients to the blood.

SIX EXOGENOUS PATHOGENIC FACTORS

Exogenous pathogenic factors can invade the body and cause disease when Chi is weak.

WIND – Master Yang Pathogen. Sudden change, upward and outward movement, aversion to wind, trembling, tremors, seizures, dizziness, influenza, spontaneous sweating. Combines with other pathogens.

COLD – Yin Pathogen. Deficient heat, aversion to cold, contraction, coagulation, muscle spasm, slow moving, stagnation, fatigue, diarrhea, body secretions are thin, clear, profuse, pale tongue, slow pulse.

FIRE/HEAT – Yang Pathogen. Upward movement of heat, aversion to heat, thirsty, fever, headache, dark scanty urine, infection, mania, internal bleeding, red tongue, rapid pulse.

DAMP – Yin Pathogen. Downward movement, heaviness, phlegm, chronic, body aches, deficient heat, aversion to cold, coagulation, muscle spasm, slow moving, diarrhea, slow pulse.

DRY – Yang Pathogen. Lack of moisture, dryness of mouth, eyes, nose, skin, coat, lungs, and scanty urine.

SUMMER HEAT – Yang Pathogen. Only occurs during summer, upward and dispersing movement, high fever, sweating, loss of consciousness, dry tongue, dark scanty urine, extreme thirst, dehydration, shortness of breath. Often seen with dampness, causing loose stools, vomiting, and respiratory distress.

The process the TCM practitioner uses to ascertain what type of chi is not functioning is known as "distinguishing patterns of disharmony." When there's a harmonious flow of chi and blood throughout the horse's body, all is well. His internal organs are balanced and able to perform their jobs, and the horse's immune system can withstand any internal stress or external invasion. When there's a disruption to the harmonious flow of chi and blood, a pattern of disharmony becomes evident.

Let's look at chi a bit more closely to understand disruptions in the flow of chi. Chi can become stagnant and encapsulated as in the case of tumors. Chi that's supposed to descend, such as Lung chi, can ascend, which results in coughing. Stomach chi is supposed to help food substances move through and down the trachea. When Stomach chi doesn't descend, the horse can choke. Choking is known as "rebellious chi."

Each organ system has its own chi. The internal organs must perform specific tasks within the body. For instance, if Heart chi is experiencing an imbalance, it can't circulate nourishing, warming chi and blood to the other internal organs and tissues. The horse's legs could feel cold, he could be lethargic, and his eyes might be dull. When Bladder chi is imbalanced, the horse could be incontinent. When the Large Intestine chi isn't balanced, the horse may colic.

Now what does imbalance mean? What exactly is not in balance? How does an imbalance occur? The answers to these questions lie in understanding the theory of yin-yang, which is addressed in the next chapter.

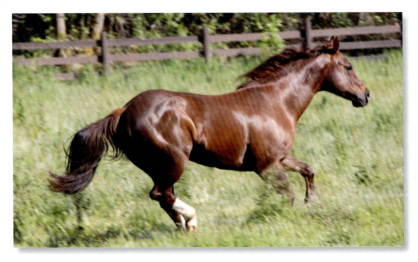

Chapter Five

THEORY OF YIN-YANG

The ancient Chinese were highly connected to the natural cycles of life, days, and seasons. They understood that the crops would grow abundantly in the summer when they received enough light and warmth of the sun during the day and the dark, coolness, and damp of night. It takes the balance of both day and night to produce a good crop.

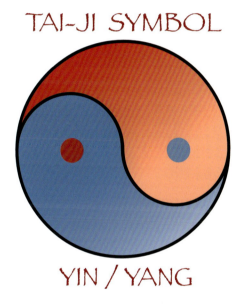

TAI-JI SYMBOL

YIN / YANG

When the hot sun beats down for long summer days and there's little rain to nourish the growing sprouts, the crops dry up and wither in the field. If too many cloudy, rainy days occur, the opposite happens; the soil becomes saturated and the crops rot. This imbalance of too much or too little sun and heat leads to a lack of food and the ability to sustain life. Everything in nature, including the living body, must have the balance of day and night, heat and cool, dry and wet to thrive.

Yin and yang are the two dynamic forces that constitute chi. Combined, these two opposing, yet interdependent, forces are the difference between life and death. Yin and yang make up the one entity called chi.

Nature of Yin and Yang

Yin and yang are labels for a specific set of characteristics or attributes. Yin is associated with water and all the attributes of water such as wet, cold, flowing downward, and nourishing. Yang is exactly opposite. Yang is associated with fire, which is dry and hot, rises, and is consuming.

Yang is like Fire	Yin is like Water
Hot	Cold
Active	Slow
Dry	Wet
Action is upward	Action is downward
Red (Light)	Blue or Black (Dark)
Consumes	Nourishes
Lacks density	Has substance

When your horse is full of zestful energy, he is acting more yang in nature. When your elderly mare is nodding off in the shade of a tree, she is being more yin in nature. If you've been riding on a hot day and your gelding has not had access to water for a while, he could become dehydrated, which is more yang in nature. Dehydration indicates too much yang. Perhaps you arrive at a cool stream and your horse drinks and drinks lots of water and becomes overly hydrated, resulting in too much water, or too much yin.

Horses are constantly balancing themselves. On hot, sunny days, most horses will seek cooling shade and water when they've had enough heat. On cold windy days, horse will stand closer to each other for warmth and seek shelter from the wind. This balancing process is obvious in external equine behavior; however, this same process is going on internally at all times.

On The Body

Yin	Yang
Foot	Head
Chest / Abdomen	Spine / Back
Female	Male
Interior of body	Surface of body
Older	Younger

Temperament

Yin	Yang
Withdrawn	Outgoing
Timid	Aggressive
Quiet	Loud
Low activity	Highly active
Calm	Anxious
Relaxed	Energetic
Gentle	Rough

On Earth

Yin	Yang
Water	Fire
Cold	Hot
Wet	Dry
Earth	Heaven
Moon	Sun
Night	Day
Winter	Summer
Below	Above
Dark	Light

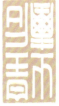

Circulation of blood throughout the animal's body is associated with yang because it's the movement of blood. Blood itself is considered yin in nature because it's fluid and nourishing. The yang activity of circulating blood and the yin nature of the blood itself work together to warm and nourish the internal organs, bones, muscles, and other tissues. For chi to flow harmoniously throughout the horse's body, yin and yang must be in constant dynamic balance.

Pattern of Harmony

When yin and yang are in relative balance, chi is flowing harmoniously. When chi is actively nourishing his body, your horse is healthy. His immune system is functioning optimally. He's the four-legged definition of equine vitality.

Think of all the good things a healthy horse portrays. When yin and yang are in balance, his internal organs can function properly because they're receiving chi, blood, and other vital substances needed. His coat is dappled and shiny. His muscles are beautifully defined and full. He's alert and his eye is bright. He moves with confidence. He's happy in his herd and enjoys the company of humans. His entire being emanates vigor and joy. This healthy horse evinces what Chinese medicine calls a pattern of harmony.

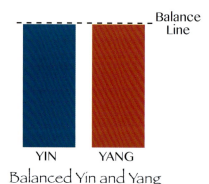

Balanced Yin and Yang

This image depicts yin and yang being equal. Notice both yin and yang are touching the balance line.

Four Patterns of Disharmony

A pattern of disharmony occurs when yin and yang are not in balance. If there's too much or too little of either yin or yang, this imbalance can lead to disease. Learning how these patterns appear provides you with a way of assessing and balancing your horse. TCM delineates four basic patterns of disharmony: Excess Yang, Excess Yin, Deficient Yang, and Deficient Yin.

Excess Patterns of Disharmony

In general, excess patterns tend to be acute in nature. More often than not, they occur in younger rather than older horses. Excess patterns are short-lived and considered superficial because they don't penetrate deeply into the body and cause tissue damage. With excess patterns, the horse will recover relatively quickly and most likely be restored to complete health.

1. **Excess yang pattern.** When there's an excess of yang, there's less yin to balance it. The horse could be feverish, manifest manic behavior, or lose weight suddenly—indicators of an excess yang condition or heat syndrome. The horse's tongue may be red and his pulse could feel rapid, even bounding.

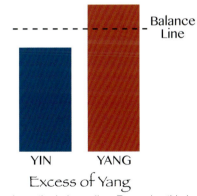

Excess of Yang
Yang chi is above the balance line. To resolve this heat condition, the excess yang needs to be dispersed.

In TCM, the way to deal with excess yang conditions is to disperse the heat get rid of the excess yang chi. By reducing the excess yang chi, yang goes back to the balance line. Then yin can come back to the balance line because yang is no longer consuming it.

Picture this: Your horse is upset and anxiously running up and down the fence line for hours because you moved his best friend to another paddock. He won't even stop to take a drink from the water trough. By the end of the day, he's overwrought, hot, sweaty, and dehydrated. This presents an example of a yang excess pattern of disharmony. You make sure he drinks water and reunite him with his best buddy and, by the next morning, your horse is calm, cool, and collected, grazing alongside his friend as if yesterday never happened. The heat of anxiety and dehydration is resolved, and your horse can happily resume his yin-yang balance with no permanent damage.

2. **Excess yin pattern.** When there's an excess of yin, too much wet and/or cold, a horse can suddenly be weak and lethargic, feel cold to the touch, have diarrhea, and seem achy because she doesn't want to move around. Other indicators of an excess yin pattern include a pale tongue and slow pulse.

Maybe there's been a sudden cold snap and it's as if the cold has invaded the horse's body. Or the horse consumes a huge amount of cold water and feels bloated and achy. Most yin excesses are a result of external cold invading the body.

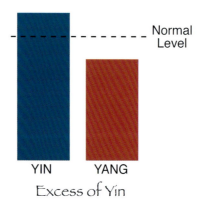

Excess of Yin

Yin chi is above the balance line. To resolve this cold condition, the cold must be dispersed.

Note that yang has been consumed by the excess yin. Whenever either yin or yang is in excess (above the balance line), the other is being consumed. To rebalance the yin excess, the cold needs to be dispersed.

Say you're on an easy-going trail ride and the temperature suddenly drops, clouds form, and it rains. You make your way back to your farm, and when you're walking your horse back to her stall, you notice she's cold, wet, and shivering. This is an excess yin pattern of disharmony. You need to help her get rid of the cold by walking her until her coat dries and her body is warm again. Excess cold syndromes are short-term and easy to resolve, with no permanent damage to the horse's body.

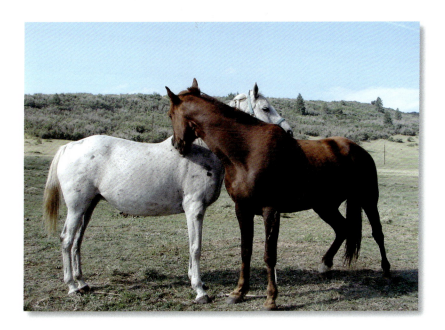

Deficient Patterns of Disharmony

Deficient patterns are chronic in nature; they've taken a long time to manifest. These patterns usually present in older horses and cannot be fully resolved. Once a long-term, deficient condition occurs, it likely requires ongoing management because some form of tissue or energetic damage has taken place. Not everything can be "fixed"; a chronic health problem is exactly that, chronic.

3. **Deficient yang pattern.** This pattern is considered a cold pattern because there's not enough heat chi (yang chi) to balance the cold chi (yin chi). Thus yang is below the balance line. That means there's too little heat or activity present to balance the cold, which is up to the normal balance line. The condition only appears cold because there's not enough heat.

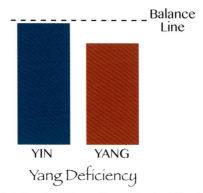

Yang chi is below the balance line, while yin chi is at the balance line. To manage this condition, yang chi needs to be "tonified" or stimulated to bring yang back up to the balance line.

The yang deficiency pattern is often called Empty Cold or False Cold because it seems like a cold syndrome but it's only cold because the body isn't generating enough heat to balance the cold. Indicators of a yang deficiency include sores that aren't healing, poor appetite, on-going digestion issues, consistent shortness of breath, and chronic exhaustion. The horse's pulse might feel slow and weak; his tongue might be pale and swollen or puffy.

The yang deficiency imbalance can be managed by stimulating, also called tonifying, the yang chi. This is achieved by using acupoints known to increase the heat in the body and enhance chi circulation. Odds are, because of age or injury, the issue won't be completely resolved. However, the horse can regain her spunk and be much more comfortable by bringing up her yang chi.

Ever have a 24-year old mare who felt she was too old to go for an easy trail ride? Did she just stand around in the paddock resting one leg after the other, sleeping on and off, not grazing with enthusiasm? Well, after a few acupressure sessions to enhance her yang chi, she just might be reinvigorated and ready for anything!

4. **Deficient yin pattern.** This pattern is a heat pattern because there's not enough cold yin to balance the heat of yang. Yang is at the balance line; yin is below balance. When there's not enough cold to balance, the animal will appear hot. A horse can feel warm to the touch, seem restless or agitated, be consistently dehydrated, become emaciated, and experience muscle atrophy (loss of muscle tissue). Two other indicators of a yin deficiency are a rapid yet weak pulse and pale red tongue.

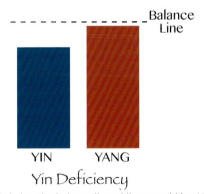

Yin Deficiency

Yin chi is below the balance line while yang chi is at the balance line. To manage this condition, yin chi needs to be "tonified," or stimulated, to bring yin back up to the balance line.

This yin deficiency pattern of disharmony is also called Empty Heat or False Heat as it only appears or feels like a heat syndrome because there's not enough of the cooling and/or substantive nature of yin. Remember, some form of yin chi has sustained damage and cannot fully recover. The TCM practitioner can use acupoints to help restore the balance of yin by tonifying yin, but because it's a chronic condition, supporting yin becomes a consistent objective.

As horses age, they tend to lose muscle mass because the muscles aren't able to absorb nutrients the way they did when they were younger. Some people call this natural aging process "senior wasting." In TCM terms, it's considered a yin deficiency because the horse is not able to sustain his body substance. Acupressure can help maintain the fullness of the muscles for as long as possible.

In summary, the Theory of Chi along with the Theory of Yin-Yang are the two most ancient theories underlying Chinese medicine. Chi can warm, nourish, protect, and control bodily functions when yin and yang are in dynamic balance.

Providing your horse with a healthy, natural lifestyle definitely contributes to his longevity. And, like all of Chinese medicine, acupressure is a preventive form of healthcare, so by adding acupressure to his regime, you can support an even greater quality of life for your horse.

Chapter Six

FIVE-ELEMENT THEORY

The Five-Element Theory came much later than the Theories of Chi and Yin-Yang. Like the other theories underlying Chinese Medicine, it was derived from Taoist philosophy.

In Chinese, the Five Elements are called *Wu Zing*. *Wu* means five, while *Zing* can be translated as "movement, change, transition, transformation, or process" in English. Thus, the original conceptual intent was to refer to the idea of Five Phases of Transformation also seen as The Five Phases of Transition. In the West, it's common to refer to these five phases, or movements, as "elements" because they're identified by five basic constituents of nature: Wood, Fire, Earth, Metal, and Water.

One of the earliest direct references to the Five-Element Theory appeared during the Western Han Dynasty (206 BC–AD 24) in a book titled *Great Transmission of the Valued Book*, which reads, "Water and Fire provide food, Metal and Wood provide prosperity and the Earth makes provisions." This reference initiated the view of the five elements as they relate to human survival. Zou Yan (c. 350–270 BC), who was part of the Naturalist School, provided some insights into the original thinking behind the development of the Five-Element Theory in this statement: "Each of the five elements is followed by one it cannot conquer."

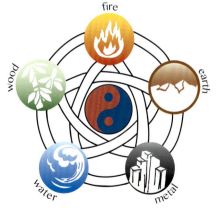

Prior to the Five-Element Theory, illness was attributed to evil spirits and other supernatural causes that would descend upon a poor suffering animal or human. The Five-Element Theory, when applied to Chinese medicine, provided and continues to provide a more "scientific" method of distinguishing imbalances leading to disease. This theory serves as a model

> **"The Five Phases are water, fire, wood, metal, and earth. Water moistens and flows downward. Fire flares upward. Wood flexes. Metal can be transformed by casting. And earth serves for the planting and growing of crops."**
>
> — General Regulations, *The Book of History*

or construct by which deductive and inductive thought is used to understand the nature of patterns of disease.

The Five-Element Theory established a logical connection between the natural environment and life where none had existed before. The ancient Chinese looked at the universe and all that exists and saw that everything is related to everything else. Crops cannot grow without the balance of hot sun, water, and cool nights. Humans and animals cannot live healthfully without nourishment derived from rice and other grain that grows on earth.

The Five-Element Theory is based on a deep understanding of the interrelatedness of the heavens and life on earth. All natural phenomena must be in a dynamic state of balance for there to be health of all living things, which includes the earth itself.

Balance and the Five Elements

The ancient Chinese recognized that the entire universe is constantly changing and transforming and so is a living body. The Five-Element Theory provides a conceptual model demonstrating how the internal organ systems interact and maintain a continuous, harmonious balance of yin and yang. Additionally, it provides techniques for restoring the dynamic equilibrium of yin and yang when they're not balanced. And using the Five-Element Theory to classify information gives us a powerful tool for assessment and therapeutic action.

Each element represents distinct qualities, characteristics, and properties reflected in nature. For the living body to function healthfully in the constantly changing environment, the body must continuously adapt and transition from one phase of the day, year, life-cycle, climate, etc. to the next. The body must be able to continuously transform itself to maintain a dynamic balance of yin and yang so chi can function smoothly.

Correspondences of the Elements

Wood Element. The ancient Chinese used the constituents of nature to represent the physical properties and energetic attributes of each "element." For instance, Wood represents birth and rebirth because both tend to occur in the spring; hence Wood is associated with spring. It takes an amazing amount of energy to give birth or have a seed germinate and break through the soil in the spring; thus, Wood is associated with the exuberant, ascending chi of birth and spring. For young saplings to survive the strong winds of spring, their branches need to be flexible and bend without breaking. Similarly, flexibility in the living body depends on the tensile strength of tendons and ligaments; thus, tendons and ligaments are the bodily tissue associated with Wood.

Wood is a metaphor representing spring, birth/rebirth, flexibility, fresh green, cleansing wind, powerful ascending energy, and a host of other associations and correspondences grouped together. In a similar manner, the ancient Chinese classified everything on earth, environmental cyclic transformation, and even the entire solar system.

The Liver organ system, which is considered the yin organ related to the Wood element, is responsible for the harmonious flow of chi. When there's a harmonious flow of chi, the horse's emotional state is well balanced. When the spring winds blow to clear the environment of dead wood, it can cause a disruption to the flow of chi leading to anger and irritation.

The emotion that corresponds with Wood is anger because the Liver's bile, which is produced internally, is like internal wind. When internal wind occurs, Liver yang chi can rise, leading to anger, with the heat of anger ascending to the chest and head. The sense orifice associated with Wood is the eye which corresponds with eyes becoming red and watery when spring winds blow. Also, if the Liver isn't healthy, the eyes can become jaundiced.

All of the correspondences with Wood are in some way related to the properties of Wood in a poetic form. Trees have green leaves, so the color associated with Wood is green. The sense organ of Wood are the eyes, so tears are often considered the "fluid" of Wood. In some texts, bile is the fluid of Wood because the Liver produces bile. Nails are seen as an extension of the tendon concept and an outward manifestation of the health of the Liver. After thousands of years of observation, a definite correlation has been established between the health of the nails and the health of the Liver.

Fire Element. Each element represents a host of different energies and attributes. Fire energy is expansive and rises. The season of Fire is summer, the hottest time of the annual cycle. Because summer is the season of the greatest growth, the life-cycle stage of Fire is growth. The color associated with Fire is red because it's the hottest color. The main yin organ system for the Fire element is the Heart, "Monarch of the Body," which is responsible for the fair apportionment and circulation of blood which warms and nourishes all parts of the body. The emotion of Fire is joy, which positively and dramatically affects the Heart function.

When a horse is balanced in the Fire Element, he usually enjoys life and gets along with his herd and humans alike. He is probably an amazing athlete because his vascular system is working well throughout his body.

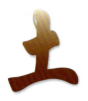

Earth Element. The Earth produces food to nourish the body. The Stomach and Spleen organ systems are responsible for holding and creating bio-absorbable nutrients; hence they're the organs associated with Earth. The energy of Earth is stabilizing and is thought of as the center; it's the balance of yin and yang chi.

In Chinese thought, there are five season, not four. The fifth season is late summer when the crops mature, which corresponds with the bounty of Earth. The emotion associated with the Earth element is worry or overthinking. When animals are worried, their appetite and digestion may be disrupted. When horses are grazing, they're usually calm and feeling centered and grounded on earth. The mouth is the sensory orifice associated with Earth because grazing is related to the mouth.

Muscles are the parts of the body governed by the Spleen and Stomach. When the body is well nourished, muscles can function properly; when it's not well nourished, muscles can atrophy. A horse balanced in the Earth element is a contented, solid mount that takes good care of his rider.

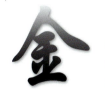

Metal Element. Metal energy is contracting, like the in-gathering of the harvest in autumn. The emotion of Metal is grief because grief causes the body to contract. In fact, the walls of the Lung actually thicken and contract during times of grief or sorrow. The *zang-fu* (internal) organs of the Metal element are the Lung and Large Intestine. Both organ systems gather chi. The Lung gathers chi (*Zong Chi*) while the Large Intestine gathers waste for expulsion. Both the Lung and Large Intestine do their job of ridding the body of toxins. These organs are responsible for releasing toxins from the body just the way we all must move on from grief or we'll become "stuck" or toxic.

The Metal element is related to middle age when life is no longer expansive but rather a time of collecting the resources already created. A horse balanced in the Metal Element is more comfortable with routine and structure.

Water Element. The Water Element is related to the cold of winter, when it's necessary to conserve energy. Horses find shelter during dark, cold winter days and nights. Human and animal energy turns inward. This element is related to old age and the end of a cycle. The Kidney and Bladder organ systems correspond with Water because they're both involved with the water metabolism of the body. Kidney governs bones because bones are the core of the body and water relates to willpower, which also reflects core strength.

Fear is the emotion associated with Water. The horse's entire survival is dependent on his ability to respond quickly to a predatory animal or a dangerous situation. The horse balanced in the Water element appears self-sufficient and resilient—a true survivor.

It's easy for our Western minds to forget how to see ourselves as an integral part of the natural environment, yet the ancient Chinese saw nothing else. Their vocabulary for medical and philosophical thought and writing was a reflection of what they saw, felt, and knew by being part of the natural flow of life. These elements or phases of change reflect both metaphor and reality. The ancient Chinese passed down a true understanding of the words Wood, Fire, Earth, Metal, and Water with all their energetic and lyric qualities.

Take time to carefully review the Correspondence Chart on the following page. It becomes more meaningful the more you meditate on each of the associations in relation to an element. At times, you need to suspend rational thought and allow your mind to flow into a more poetic frame of mind to gain a deeper understanding of the phases of transformation.

Five-Element Theory Cycles

According to the Five-Element Theory, the natural world includes two clear cycles, or natural movements, associated with having the elements in balance. They are:

- The Creation, or *Sheng*, cycle, represents building, growth, and promoting.
- The Control, or *Ko*, cycle balances the Creation cycle by inhibiting and restraining growth.

If no force existed to check Creation, there would be exponential growth, which could be highly destructive and extremely unbalanced. A Control cycle must exist to avoid an over-abundance of growth, and a Growth Cycle must exist to avoid over-control. The two cycles balance each other the way yin and yang dynamically create and consume each other.

For instance, if water didn't extinguish fire, everything would burn and the world would be ravaged by fire. Or, if a horse were exposed to extreme cold for days on end and he became hypothermic and could not regain heat in his body, he would die.

FIVE PHASES OF TRANSFORMATION CORRESPONDENCE CHART

	METAL	WATER	WOOD	FIRE	EARTH
ENERGY	Contracting	Conserving	Generative	Expansive	Stabilizing
YIN-YANG PHASE	New Yin	Full Yin	New Yang	Full Yang	Yin-Yang Balance
TRANSITION / LIFE CYCLE	Harvest / Middle Age	Storage / Old Age to Death	Birth	Creation / Growth	Maturity
SEASON	Fall	Winter	Spring	Summer	Late Summer
CLIMATE	Dry/Wind	Cold	Windy	Hot	Wet/Humid
DIRECTION	West	North	East	South	Center
COLOR	White	Blue	Green	Red	Yellow
EMOTION	Grief	Fear	Anger	Joy	Sympathy/Worry
SENSORY ORIFICE	Nose	Genitals/Ears	Eyes	Tongue	Mouth
SMELL	Rotten	Putrid	Rank	Burning	Fragrant/Sweet
GOVERNED PART OF BODY	Skin & Body Hair	Bones & Marrow	Tendons & Ligaments	Vascular System	Muscles & Lymph
MERIDIANS	Lung & Large Intestine	Kidney & Bladder	Liver & Gall Bladder	Heart & Sm Intestine Pericardium & Triple Heater	Spleen & Stomach

Too much of *anything* can be disastrous. Conversely, too much control of anything can be equally horrific. The natural world of checks and balances results in a healthy balance. Both the Creation cycle and Control cycle are absolutely necessary.

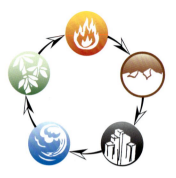

CREATION CYCLE

Wood creates Fire
Fire creates Earth
Earth creates Metal
Metal creates Water
Water creates Wood

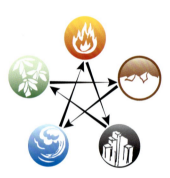

CONTROL CYCLE

Fire controls Metal
Earth controls Water
Metal controls Wood
Wood controls Earth
Water controls Fire

In the diagram depicting the five elements and their interrelationships, the Creation cycle flows in a clockwise direction and the movement of the Control cycle takes the form of a five-pointed star. Looking at the diagram, note that Wood creates Fire because wood fuels fire; and, Water controls Fire because water puts out Fire. In turn, Fire controls Metal since the heat of fire melts metal. Metal controls Wood because the sharp edge of a metal tool cuts wood.

This is how the elements balance each other naturally. Ideally, there should be no excess or deficiency of growth and no overly extended control or lack of control within the forces that govern the functioning of the body.

Often, the relationships of the elements are described as part of a family. The first relationship of the creation cycle is the mother to son, or child, relationship. The mother is the creator of the element that follows. In other words, Wood is the mother of Fire, Fire is the mother of Earth, Earth is the mother of Metal, and Metal is the mother of Water.

Looking at this relationship from the opposite side, Fire is considered the child, or son, of Wood, Earth is the child of Fire, Metal is the child of Earth, and so on. This family analogy gets more complicated when taken to the next level of relationship in the Creation cycle by calling Earth the grandchild of Wood, Metal the grandchild of Fire, and so on. Using this family analogy is important for understanding the mindset of the ancient Chinese as well as differentiating patterns.

As a conceptual model for balancing yin and yang, the Five-Element Theory depicts the interrelationships of the internal organ systems. Each of the paired internal organs is associated with a specific element. For Instance, Stomach and Spleen correspond with the Earth element, and Lung and Large Intestine correspond with the Metal element. According to this theory, Earth creates Metal. Given the family analogy, Earth is the mother of Metal, which denotes the relationship between Earth and Metal. It's also stating a relationship between Stomach/Spleen and Lung/Large Intestine—the Earth paired organs create the Metal paired organs.

Say there's deficient yang chi in the Lung organ system, which is in the Metal element. The mother of Metal is Earth and the mother can nourish the child. By using acupoints known to tonify Earth yang chi, you are helping to nourish the Lung organ system. This is the way each of the internal organs can help each other restore balance. The interrelationships of the organ systems can be simple and yet become more complicated, but the basic premise of balance is always the intention.

Differentiating Patterns

Because the Five-Element Theory helps to classify information, it provides a framework for assessing your horse's current condition. The correspondences for each element offer a resource for readily identifying a pattern of disharmony.

If your horse were exhibiting a watery nasal discharge and excess mucus in his throat and chest, a TCM practitioner would say he's suffering from an Invasion of Cold (or Excess Yin condition—also known as the common cold). All the indicators are associated with the Lung, hence it's a Metal Pattern of Disharmony. This provides an understanding of how to approach the Lung imbalance.

Here's another example: Your horse's hooves are dry, chipped, and somewhat painful, causing him to walk more gingerly than usual. Hooves, like human nails, are related to the Liver organ system, and Liver is the yin organ associated with the Wood element. Hence, your horse has a Wood imbalance.

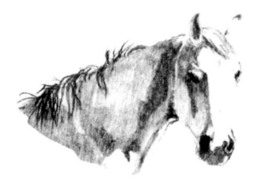

Understanding the Five Elements can provide a shorthand method of grasping the complexities of your horse's health issue. It's highly insightful and helps to identify and isolate specific conditions and tendencies your horse might have. Like all TCM theories, the Five-Element Theory is another tool in distinguishing patterns of disharmony and resolving the imbalance of yin and yang, thus restoring the harmonious flow of chi throughout the horse's body.

Yin-Yang Theory and the Five-Element Theory are central to Traditional Chinese Medicine. Both are simple and poetic in reflecting the nature of everything that exists. On the other hand, both theories lead to increasing levels of detail and sophistication and can become highly complex.

Chapter Seven

Zang-fu and Meridian Theory

The *Zang-Fu* and Meridian Theory is the core of Eastern pathology. *Zang-Fu* refers to the internal organs. Meridians are the channels or pathways along which the chi of the internal organs travels throughout the horse's (or person's) body. Together, the internal *zang-fu* organs and the meridians are considered complete organ systems.

In Chinese Medicine, the concept of the internal organs is quite different from the current conventional Western medicine concept. Though the organs have the same names as they do in Western medicine, in talking about an organ system, the Chinese approach refers to all the functions and attributes ascribed to the organ system. It's a bigger conceptual model. To make this readily apparent, the first letter of the organ is capitalized, and the name of the organ is spoken of in the singular.

For example, in TCM, Lung is not just involved in respiration, though that's one of its primary functions. Lung includes the descending and dispersing of chi, creates and stores Chest chi (*Zong* chi), circulates Defensive chi, and controls skin and skin hair; plus grief is the emotion associated with Lung, to name just a few of the Lung's role within the body.

When referring to a *zang-fu* organ, or internal organ, we're relating to a bigger picture that's a dynamic, energetic entity with many attributes, including an emotion, direction of chi flow, sensory orifice, type of body fluid, bodily tissue, production and storage of a vital substance, time of day for optimal chi flow, and so on.

Each *zang-fu* organ has its own yin and yang chi that needs to be in dynamic balance for it to function properly and carry out all of its work to maintain a harmonious flow of chi. All of the organ systems are dependent on each other for the horse's body to be healthy.

It's exactly these ideas that make Chinese medicine fascinating and a bit difficult for the western mind to grasp. Just sit with these notions and allow them to be suspended in your consciousness while you gather more and more information to mull. You'll likely experience many "aha" moments as you continue to study. Things will fall into place in your mind because the theories and concepts are based on the natural flow of life and the interdependence of everything.

Zang-Fu Theory

The internal organs are called the *zang-fu* organs, while the theory of the *zang-fu* organs is called *Zang Xiang*. *Zang* refers to the internal location of the organs while *Xiang* connotes the manifestation or reflective image of the organs. Referring to the manifestation of the organs brings us back to the Law of Integrity. The Law of Integrity states that what occurs internally can be seen externally on the body.

When the *zang-fu* organs function properly, you see no outward manifestations of an imbalance; your horse looks and acts like a healthy animal. When the *zang-fu* organs are not in balance thus not able to function optimally, you see indicators on the surface of the body or in the horse's behavior, letting you know all is not well.

Zang organs are the core yin organs. Most texts identify five *zang* organs: Lung, Heart, Spleen, Liver, and Kidney. Some texts include the Pericardium, the sac surrounding and protecting the Heart, as a yin organ and some don't. That's why you will see a discrepancy in there being five or six yin organs identified at times.

In general, the *zang* organs create and store vital substances, which include chi, blood, essence, *shen* (consciousness / spirit), and body fluids. The *zang* organs, hidden deep in the trunk of the body, are solid in form.

Fu organs are the yang organs. The *fu* organs are yang in nature because their chief role is to transport substances such as food, water, and waste. The yang organs are not considered to be as deep in the body as the yin organs. Five of these six organs tend to be hollow and tubular in form: Large Intestine, Stomach, Small Intestine, Bladder, and Gall Bladder. The sixth, the Triple Heater, is energetic and has no form, as explained later in this chapter.

Yin and yang organ systems are paired like husband and wife, or sisters. Yin and yang organs, like the rest of the body, need to be in balance. If the energy of one of the paired organs isn't in balance, the energy of the other can help to balance it because they are internally related.

For instance, the Lung is the yin organ system related to the Large Intestine, which is the yang organ system. When Lung is imbalanced, Large Intestine can "lend" either yin or yang chi, as needed, to help balance it. It is an on-going process in the body.

ORGAN SYSTEMS

Zang / Yin		Fu / Yang
Lung	&	Large Intestine
Spleen	&	Stomach
Heart	&	Small Intestine
Kidney	&	Bladder
Pericardium*	&	Triple Heater
Liver	&	Gall Bladder

* Some texts include the Pericardium as a yin organ; many do not. The *zang-fu* organs are typically presented as five zang organs and six fu organs. However, the Pericardium meridian is considered as significant in its function as any other meridian.

Organ Systems

The ancient Chinese were interested in how the body functioned as a whole rather than its parts in isolation. Their reasoning was clear—everything in a body is related. For example, when an animal experiences grief due to the loss of a mate, the walls of the lungs become constricted and thicken. There's an actual physiological change to the tissue. Taking a deep breath becomes difficult. Lung function becomes limited.

If the animal isn't able to move through the grief, the lungs continue to be constricted. Lung function declines and can result in respiratory disease due to stagnation of fluids in the lungs. The Lung plays a vital role in maintaining the immune system. If the Lung is compromised, the immune system becomes compromised.

The imbalance of one *zang-fu* organ can have a cascading effect on other organs. Nothing is isolated. The inability of one system to perform its role within the body can present a pathological progression of indicators. In Chinese medicine, this progression of indicators sets up a pattern of disharmony.

Addressing the interrelatedness of the organ systems provides an understanding of TCM. Eastern pathology was developed through thousands of years of observation and practical clinical experience. It describes the functions of the *zang-fu* organs, the relationships between them, and their impact on the body.

> **"Internally, the 12 major meridians connect with the *Zang-fu* organs, and externally with joints, limbs, and the other superficial tissues of the body."**
> —Huang Di and Qi Bo, *Miraculous Pivot*

Meridians

Meridian theory is based on *Zang-Fu* theory. Each meridian is connected to an internal organ. All of the attributes of the *zang-fu* organs are also ascribed to the meridian. When you're working with acupoints along the Liver meridian, you're stimulating the activities of the Liver organ as well. (You'll learn more about the 12 Major Meridians and two Extraordinary Vessels in the next chapter.)

Meridians function as energetic extensions of the internal organs. They're relatively "superficial" compared to the organs because they're located just beneath the surface of the skin. Various numbers of acupressure points, or acupoints, are located along each meridian. When stimulating acupoints, you're affecting the energy of its internal organ's function, which in turn affects the entire meridian network. Remember, organ systems are comprised of the organ itself with all its multi-functional activities plus its meridian.

Meridians can be defined as pathways or channels along which chi and blood flow to nourish the body. A vast network of meridians throughout the body supports the health of all of the organs, bones, skin, joints, muscles, hair, and processes. Together, this network of channels and collateral vessels are called *Jing Lou*.

The meridian system is a communication system that transmits and circulates energetic chi and nourishing blood (*xue*) as well as energetic information and other vital substances to all parts of the body. The 12 Major Meridians transmit information and substances from the interior *zang-fu* organs to the exterior superficial, tissues. Each *zang-fu* organ has its own functions and processes for which it's responsible. These responsibilities are carried out by their meridian.

Gall Bladder & Liver Meridians

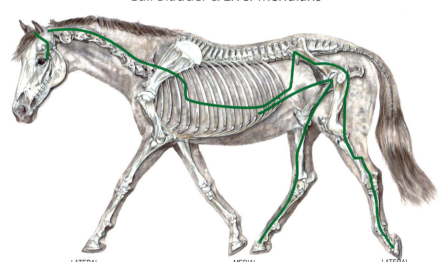

LATERAL   MEDIAL   LATERAL

As an example, the Liver organ system is the Strategic Planner of the body. It's responsible for the harmonious flow of chi among the *zang-fu* organs, replenishing the blood, making sure there's enough blood in the vessels for activity, nourishing tendons and ligaments (sinews), supplying fluids and visual acuity to the eyes, and managing the emotions so that anger doesn't disrupt the flow of chi and blood. That's a lot to do!

The yin-yang chi of the Liver organ itself generates these activities, and the Liver meridian carries out these missions. This creates the internal-external connection between the organ and the surface of the body where we can access the acupoints and influence the flow of energy and nutrients.

Meridians are responsible for the communication between the organ systems as well as the regulation of chi and blood flow for each of the organs. Each organ system receives its optimal flow, or concentration, of chi and blood for two hours during a 24-hour period. It's like a two-hour "tune-up."

Practitioners can use the time and direction of the flow of chi to assess a horse's condition and determine when an acupressure session could be most beneficial. For example, if a horse is having a problem absorbing nutrients, the practitioner can offer him an acupressure session between 9 and 11 a.m., the time when Spleen is receiving its boost of chi, to enhance the effect of the session. The Spleen is responsible for Nutrient chi.

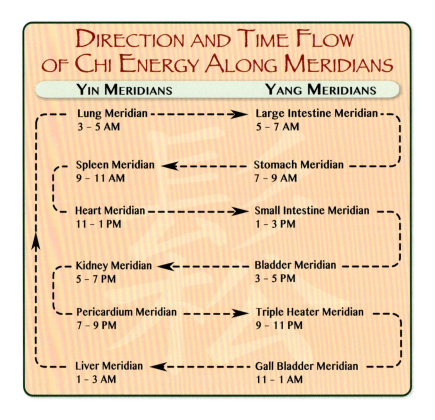

Another example: Say your horse seems agitated and restless between one and three in the morning. His behavior is indicating an imbalance in the Liver meridian. One to three in the morning is the time when Liver receives its optimal flow of chi and should be the most emotionally comfortable time for your horse. So if his behavior is agitated, check for a Liver imbalance.

The next chapter focuses on the 12 Major Meridians that connect the interior *zang-fu* organs with the exterior portions of the body. It discusses two of the eight Extraordinary Vessels, the Conception Vessel, *Ren Mai*, and the Governing Vessel, *Du Mai,* because they have their own acupressure points along them. The remaining six Extraordinary Vessels don't have acupressure points.

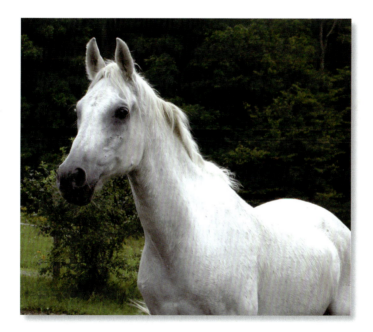

ACU-HORSE: A GUIDE TO EQUINE ACUPRESSURE

Traditional Chinese Medicine List of Concepts

Law of Integrity
   The body is a whole: What is occurring internally manifests externally

Five Stems of Chinese Medicine
   Acupuncture / Acupressure
   Tui Na (Meridian Massage)
   Diet
   Chi Gong (Exercise Technique)
   Herbs

Functions of Chi
   Promotes   Controls
   Warms   Activates
   Defends   Nourishes

Yin-Yang Theory
   Opposites
   Interdependent
   Mutually consuming
   Transform into each other
   Pattern of Disharmony –

   Excess –
      Yang: Sedate Yang
      Yin: Sedate Yin

   Deficiency –
      Yang: Tonify Yang
      Yin: Tonify Yin

Zang – Fu & Meridian Theory
   12 Major Organs / Meridians –
      Lung / Large Intestine
      Stomach / Spleen
      Heart / Small Intestine
      Bladder / Kidney
      Pericardium / Triple Heater
      Gall Bladder / Liver
      Two Extraordinary Vessels –
         Conception Vessel
         Governing Vessel

Five-Element Theory
   Wood   Earth   Water
   Fire   Metal

The Four Examinations
   Observation
   Listening / Smelling
   Questions / Inquiry
   Physical Palpation
      Association points
      Alarm points

Vital Substances
   Chi
   Blood
   Body Fluids

Eight Principles
   Exterior – Interior
   Hot – Cold
   Excess – Deficiency
   Yin – Yang

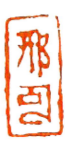

Chapter Eight

12 Major Meridians and 2 Extraordinary Vessels

To reiterate, meridians link the entire body to create a single, yet vast, network throughout your horse's body. If an organ were to fail, the entire network would fail. The meridian network is a constant interdependent, mutual support system, each organ performing its role within the system for the health of the organic whole.

Meridians and Acupressure

Meridians are the energetic reflection and distribution system of the organ system for which they're named. For example, the Lung meridian is connected internally to the horse's lungs. It flows superficially, just under the skin, from the upper thoracic region (chest) down the medial side of the forelimb to the back-inside of the horse's coronary band. This is the physical location of the Lung meridian, although the energetics and functions of the Lung extend throughout the horse's body.

Let's continue to use the Lung meridian as the example to further understand how meridians and acupoints are used in acupressure. The Lung meridian communicates with the Lung organ internally and extends the energetic functions of the Lung organ to the surface of the body. You can access the functional energetics of the Lung by working with the pools of energy known as acupoints, located along the Lung meridian. During an acupressure session, when you stimulate these acupoints, you're helping to resolve an imbalance within the Lung organ or along the Lung meridian.

For instance, when a horse tires easily and his breathing sounds raspy, you know that Lung is not balanced because it's not functioning properly. You can apply pressure to acupoints along the Lung meridian, such as Lung 7, which will begin the process of balancing the Lung. By stimulating an acupoint, you're influencing the flow of blood and chi along the Lung meridian, affecting the Lung organ as well.

ACU-HORSE: A Guide To Equine Acupressure

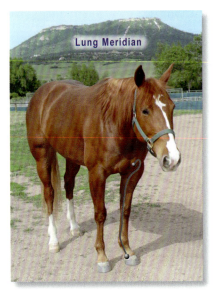

Let's go back to the physical location of the Lung meridian for a moment. Say your horse injures his carpus. You can use what are called "local points" along the Lung meridian above and below the injury to help remove toxins and replenish healthy blood and chi in the area. Because the Lung meridian runs through the horse's carpus, palpating the local points enhances the healing process.

Remember, acupoints along the meridians serve to manage imbalances related to the *zang-fu* organ system as well as address trauma or other issues that occur along the physical pathway of the meridian.

Zang-Fu Organ System Functions

Knowing the functions and energetics of the *zang-fu* organ systems is absolutely essential to being able to assess your horse's condition, or pattern of disharmony, and helping resolve the condition. Each organ system has its own associated correspondences that provide indicators of balance. By knowing the proper functioning of the organ system, you can detect an imbalance.

Because the Law of Integrity says what happens internally will manifest externally, you can see internal organ and meridian imbalances. From there, you know how to interpret them by learning the functions and energetics of each *zang-fu* organ system. This is the key to Eastern pathology.

Using the Lung as the example again, let's walk through the process to understand how the functions of the *zang-fu* organ system indicate what steps to take in restoring balance.

Indicators and Assessment. The Lung is *not* balanced when your horse exhibits respiratory issues. Remember, the Lung governs respiration. When you see a discharge from your horse's nose, you know he has an imbalance in the Lung organ system. (The orifice of the Lung is the nose, and the fluid of the Lung is mucus.)

Acupoint Selection. You can select acupoints known to enhance Lung function and restore balance. Acupoints commonly used to help resolve respiratory issues are Lung 7 and Lung 9.

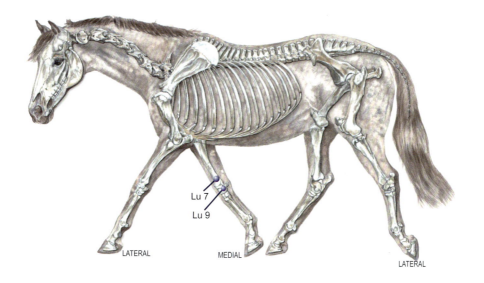

Although acupressure works by stimulating points related to the organ out of harmony, your horse may display a number of clinical signs, making assessment confusing. For simplicity's sake, focus on the indicators that are most obvious or debilitating, paying attention to the most vital issues first when figuring out how to approach your horse's condition.

In conventional veterinary medicine, any animal with an obstructed airway receives emergency care before other injuries or illnesses. In TCM, the lungs are also regarded as crucial. In Chinese medicine, the Lung stores the extremely vital substance of chi related to the breath. No breath, no life.

Because the five *zang,* or yin, organs store the vital substances and are located in the deepest layer of the body, they're regarded as the most vital organ systems. Imbalances in the *zang* organs are usually addressed first in an acupressure session. Imbalances within the *fu,* or yang, organs also need to be addressed. However, they can be seen as secondary unless there's an intestinal impaction or trauma, or other obvious emergency care is needed.

The more you study the locations, functions, and energetics of the *zang-fu* organs and their related meridians, the better you'll be able to distinguish patterns of disharmony your horse may be experiencing and address the imbalance directly.

The rest of this chapter lists the attributes of the 12 Major Meridians and 2 Extraordinary Vessels. Additionally, it includes charts and photographs depicting the flow of the meridians, along with key acupoints for each meridian.

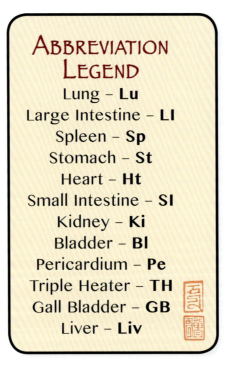

Abbreviation Legend
Lung – **Lu**
Large Intestine – **LI**
Spleen – **Sp**
Stomach – **St**
Heart – **Ht**
Small Intestine – **SI**
Kidney – **Ki**
Bladder – **Bl**
Pericardium – **Pe**
Triple Heater – **TH**
Gall Bladder – **GB**
Liver – **Liv**

"**The smooth traveling of chi and blood in the channels brings nutrients to the body, helps the balance of yin and yang, and invigorates the tendons, bones, and joints.**"

—Huang Di and Qi Bo, Treatise on the Original Organs, *Miraculous Pivot*

LUNG
Foreleg *Taiyin* /Greater Yin
Master of the Pulse

The very first independent act a foal makes is to take his first breath, and from that instant on, the Lung is in charge of the vital activities of his body. Lung, *Fei* in Chinese, is responsible for respiration. The tissues associated with the Lung are skin hair and skin, which also "breathes" and removes toxins from the body.

The Lung is known as the intermediary organ between the body and the environment because of the need to take in external oxygen; hence, of the yin organs, it's the most vulnerable to external pathogens. The Lung organ system is paired with the yang Large Intestine.

Functions and Attributes
- Governs respiration
- Governs and stores chi /vitality
- Controls the channels and blood vessels
- Controls dispersing and descending of chi
- Forms *Zong* /Chest chi
- Circulates *Wei* /Defensive chi
- Regulates water passages
- Controls the skin and coat
- Manifests in the skin and coat
- Sensory orifice is the nose
- Fluid is mucous
- Emotion is grief or sadness
- Belongs to the Metal Element
- Optimal flow of chi 3–5 AM

Health Issues
- Respiratory conditions
- Limited neck and shoulder mobility
- Lymphatic circulation problems
- Sensitivity to climate
- Skin problems /lackluster coat
- Poor immune system
- Allergies

Emotional Issue
- Chronic or long-term grief
- Compulsive behaviors
- Indifference or aloofness
- Stubbornness

Location and Flow of the Lung Meridian

The Lung meridian begins internally and surfaces in the hollow of the chest, where it meets the medial side of the forelimb in the pectoral muscle. This point is known as Lu 1. The meridian flows upward at a slight angle to the shoulder crease then down to the foreleg, and then runs along the craniomedial edge of the radius to a point just above the carpus. It flows on the medial side of the lower leg, ending just above the coronary band, approximately two-thirds the distance from the front of the hoof to the heel. There are 11 acupoints on the Lung meridian.

Lung Meridian

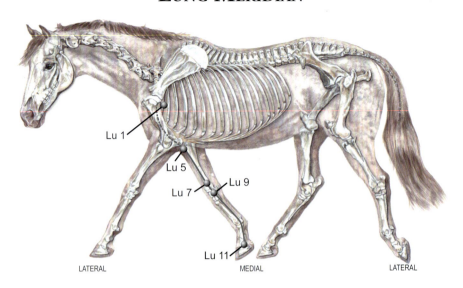

Point	Energetics/Function	Location
Lu 1	Alarm point for the Lung. Regulates and tonifies the Lungs, regulates upper Heater, and tonifies Ancestral chi. Expands and relaxes the chest, clears Heat, and stimulates the descending of Lung chi. **Benefits** any respiratory issue, shoulder, neck and back pain, or edema of the cranial thorax.	Located in the depression in the center of the muscle belly of the descending pectoral muscle at the level of the 1st intercostal space.
Lu 5	Stimulates the descending of chi, regulates and tonifies the Lungs, clears Heat. **Benefits** shoulder and elbow pain, cough or high fever.	Located on medial side of the cubital crease lateral to the tendon of the biceps trachii.
Lu 7	Connecting point, Master point for the head and neck. This point regulates the Lungs, stimulates sweating and the circulation of Protective chi, and helps to regulate the Conception Vessel. **Benefits** asthma, cough with nasal discharge, facial paralysis, deviation of the mouth and eyes, stiff neck, toothache, or issues caused by grief or sadness.	Located just cranial to the cephalic vein, at the level of the distal border of the chestnut.

Lung Meridian

Point	Energetics/Function	Location
Lu 9	Source point. Influential point for Arteries and for weakness of the pulse, and deficiency of vital energy. Regulates and tonifies the Lungs, enriches Yin, clears Heat, and promotes the redirection of rebellious chi. **Benefits** pain in the chest, asthma, cough, shoulder, and back pain, metacarpal arthritis, and laminitis.	Located in the middle of the medial aspect of the foreleg, on the radial side of the carpus, between the 1st and 2nd row of carpal bones just cranial to accessory carpal bone.
Lu 11	Jing-Well point of the Lung Meridian. Regulates the Lungs, clears Fire and Heat, and dispels Wind-Heat. Revives consciousness, calms the spirit and restores collapsed Yang. **Benefits** throat issues, respiratory problems, laminitis, sidebone, and inflammation of the heel bulbs.	Located on the caudomedial aspect of the forelimb, proximal to the coronary band.

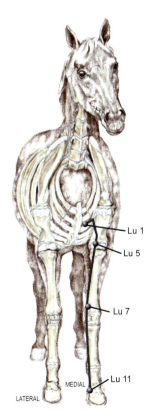

LARGE INTESTINE
Foreleg *Yangming* /Yang Brightness
The Great Eliminator

The Large Intestine, in Chinese *Da Chang*, receives food and water from the Small Intestine. It's responsible for the temporary storage of waste material and absorption of some fluid before eliminating manure. Cleansing the body of waste has both a physical and an energetic dimension. The Large Intestine plays an important part in moving stagnant chi down and out of the body. As the yang counterpart to the Lung, the Large Intestine meridian supports the respiratory and immune system functions of the Lung meridian.

Functions and Attributes
- Receives food and water from the Small Intestine
- Reabsorbs fluid, stores and excretes manure
- Descends chi
- Balances chi and blood
- Belongs to the Metal Element
- Optimal flow of chi 5–7 AM

Health Issues
- Respiratory conditions
- Mobility issues of forelimb, neck, and head
- Lymphatic circulation problems
- Sensitivity to climate
- Dental problems
- Constipation or diarrhea
- Immune system weakness
- Allergies

Emotional Issues
- Chronic or long-term grief
- Compulsive behaviors
- Indifference or aloofness
- Stubbornness
- Restlessness

Location and Flow of the Large Intestine Meridian

The Large Intestine meridian begins on the forelimb on the craniomedial side of the coronary band. It proceeds up the medial aspect of the foreleg to the carpus. It crosses laterally over the carpus and flows up the craniolateral aspect of the foreleg toward the elbow crease. It then flows up to the shoulder joint (LI 15) and across the ventral portion of the neck and on to the mandible (lower jaw). As it flows down toward the nose, it crosses on to the maxilla (upper jaw) and ends at Large Intestine 20 (LI 20) at the lateral side of the base of the nostril. There are 20 acupoints along this meridian.

Large Intestine Meridian

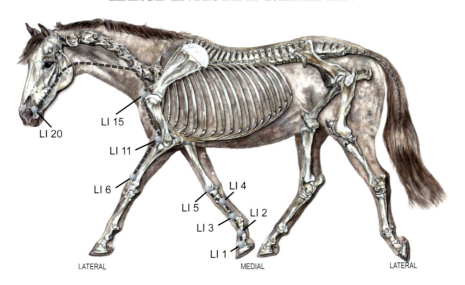

Point	Energetics/Function	Location
LI 1	Jing-Well point. Clears Lung Heat and revives consciousness. **Benefits** all hoof problems, shoulder pain or lameness of forelimb, relieves nasal discharge.	Located at the craniomedial aspect of the front hoof proximal to the coronary band.
LI 2	Clears heat, reduces swelling and alleviates pain. **Benefits** constipation or diarrhea and fever.	Found below the fetlock, in a depression cranial to the extensor branch of the suspensory ligament.
LI 3	Regulates the Large Intestine, clears Heat, and transforms Damp-Heat. **Benefits** the eyes and throat. Helps fetlock and dental pain and diarrhea or constipation.	Located above the fetlock joint, and below the medial splint bone.
LI 4	Master point for face and mouth, Source point. Alleviates exterior conditions, promotes or restrains sweating, reduces fever, helps chi flow, dispels Wind and clears Heat. Generates fluids, regulates and tonifies chi, tonifies Protective chi and alleviates pain. **Benefits** neck, forelimb, shoulder or mouth pain. Immunostimulation point, expedites labor, clears nose, opens and brightens the eyes. Restores collapsed Yang. Contraindicated in pregnancy.	Found distal and medial to the head of the medial splint bone.

Large Intestine Meridian

Point	Energetics/Function	Location
LI 5	Clears Heat and alleviates pain, calms the spirit and strengthens the sinews. **Benefits** carpal pain and dental pain.	In a depression between the 2nd and 3rd carpal bones on the craniomedial aspect of the carpus.
LI 6	Connecting point. Clears Heat, moistens dryness and dispels Wind. **Benefits** seizures, facial paralysis, upper body edema, and conjunctivitis.	Found 3 cun above LI 5 in the cranial muscle groove on the lateral aspect of the foreleg.
LI 11	Regulates Nutritive chi and blood, resolves dampness, clears Heat & alleviates itching. **Benefits** the sinews and joints, uveitis, fever, hypertension, diarrhea, and seizure.	Lateral aspect in a depression cranial to the elbow, in the transverse cubital crease.
LI 15	Relaxes the sinews, dispels Wind and clears Heat. **Benefits** shoulder pain and lameness.	Found just cranial to the point of the shoulder.
LI 20	Dispels pathogenic Heat and Wind, removes nasal obstructions. **Benefits** skin conditions, facial paralysis, colds and nasal issues, lung congestion, fatigue, and sunstroke.	Lateral to the nostril, $1/3^{rd}$ of the way down from the upper edge of the nostril.

All emergency care requires immediate veterinary attention.

STOMACH
Hind Leg *Yangming*/Yang Brightness
Sea of Nourishment

The Stomach, known in Chinese as *Wei,* is the origin of fluids and the holding basin for the "rotting and ripening" of food. The Stomach and its paired yin organ system, the Spleen, act in concert to transform food into bio-absorbable nutrients and transport them to the Heart to be converted into blood and to the Lung to be transformed into Protective chi (*Wei* chi). The nutrient-rich blood nourishes the muscles, the four limbs, and all of the body tissues. It's said that no matter what the disease, if the Stomach chi is strong, the outlook is good; conversely, if the Stomach chi is weak, the prognosis is not good.

Functions and Attributes
- Controls the "rotting and ripening" of food
- Controls the transportation of food
- Controls the descending of chi
- Contributes to Protective chi
- Originates fluids
- Tonifies chi and blood
- Belongs to the Earth Element
- Optimal flow of chi 7–9 AM

Health Issues
- Muscle tone or strength
- Digestive disorders (Colic)
- Weight problems
- Stifle problems
- Abdominal distention
- Lethargy and low stamina
- TMJ tension and pain
- Unruly appetite
- Eye problems

Emotional Issues
- Anxiety, chronic nervous tension
- Excessive worry
- Lack of focus or awareness
- Overprotective behaviors
- Obsessive behaviors

Location and Flow of the Stomach Meridian

Stomach 1 is located just below the midpoint of the eye. The meridian descends and curves around the edge of the lips and travels along the side of the jawbone, swings up the jaw in front of the ear then dives down below the cervical vertebrae. The meridian continues its flow between the front legs and travels along the mammary line to the end of the horse's ribs and into the loin area. It passes over the front aspect of the thigh and stifle, over the tibia and pastern and ends on the coronary band just lateral to the midline of the hoof at Stomach 45.

Stomach Meridian

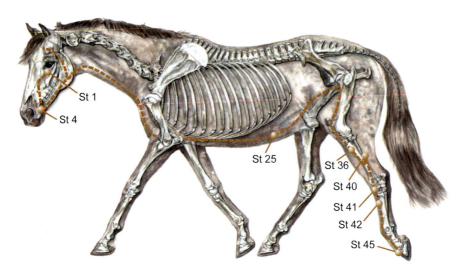

Point	Energetics/Function	Location
St 1	Brightens the eyes, dispels Wind, and clears Heat. **Benefits** conjunctivitis, uveitis, swelling, or facial paralysis.	Located directly below (ventral to) the center of the pupil.
St 4	Dispels Wind and Cold, relaxes the sinews. **Benefits** excessive salivation, eyelid tremors, dental pain, or facial paralysis.	Found at the lateral corner of the mouth.
St 25	Alarm point of the Large Intestine. Regulates the Spleen, Stomach and middle and lower Heaters. Regulates the Intestines, generates Fluids, tonifies Nutritive chi, reduces digestive stagnation, regulates chi & blood. **Benefits** gastrointestinal disorders, abdominal masses, diarrhea or constipation and edema.	Located 2 cun lateral to the umbilicus.

Stomach Meridian

Point	Energetics/Function	Location
St 36	Master point for the abdomen and GI tract. Regulates, strengthens and tonifies the Spleen, regulates the Stomach, tonifies Nutritive chi, reduces digestive stagnation, and drains pathogenic influences from the Stomach. Regulates and tonifies the Lungs. Regulates and tonifies chi and blood. Restores collapsed Yang, tonifies Protective chi. **Benefits** stomach ulcers, gastritis, lack of appetite, colic, or abdominal distension. Benefits asthma or cough. Benefits chronic consumptive disorders, allergies, anemia or generalized weakness. Benefits mastitis, constipation, and diarrhea. Useful for conditions of hypertension, seizures, shock, anxiety, fatigued extremities, and lower back pain. Contraindicated in pregnancy.	Found one half cun lateral to the tibial crest on the lateral side of the tibia.
St 40	Influential point for Phlegm, Connecting point. Regulates the Stomach and Intestines, drains pathogenic influences from the Lungs. Calms the spirit. **Benefits** Phlegm issues, edema, seizure, constipation, lower limb pain, swelling, or atrophy. Benefits fatigued extremities.	Located 8 cun proximal to the lateral malleolus, between the long and lateral digital extensors, on the lateral aspect of the hind leg.
St 41	Regulates circulation of chi, removes obstructions and eases pain. **Benefits** hock pain and abdominal disorders.	At the level of the bottom edge of lateral malleolus, between long and lateral digital extensor tendon.
St 42	Source point. Regulates the Stomach, calms the spirit, dispels Wind. **Benefits** muscular atrophy, weakness & pain of hoof, hock pain and abdominal disorders.	Located distal to the hock joint on the craniolateral aspect of the metatarsus.
St 45	Jing-Well point. Regulates Stomach, and clears Heat. **Benefits** abdominal pain, tooth pain, fever, epilepsy, or dental pain.	Located just lateral to the cranial midline of the hind hoof proximal to the coronary band.

Spleen
Hind Leg *Taiyin* /Greater Yin
Controller of Distribution

The yin organ system of the Spleen, along with the Stomach, is considered the "center within the body" and is essential to the creation of Acquired chi. It is also referred to as Post-Natal or Post-Heavenly chi, Acquired chi is necessary to sustain the horse's life after birth.

The Spleen, called *Pi* in Chinese, transforms and transports refined food essence up to combine with *Zong* /Chest chi and be converted into *Ying*/ Nutrient chi, which is even further refined to become True chi. The pure, highly-refined True chi enriches blood. If the Spleen is not functioning properly, the entire body can suffer from lack of nourishment, leading to chi and blood deficiency.

Functions and Attributes
- Governs transformation and transportation of food essence
- Controls the blood within the vessels
- Source of chi and blood
- Nourishes the muscles and four limbs
- Holds the internal organs in place
- Manifests in the lips
- Sensory orifice is the mouth
- Fluid is saliva
- Emotion is worry or over-thinking
- Belongs to the Earth Element
- Optimal flow of chi 9–11 AM

Health Issues
- Lack of muscle tone or strength
- Digestive disorders (Colic)
- Weight problems
- Stifle problems
- Pain of the medial aspect of the stifle
- Abdominal distention
- Organ prolapse
- Edema /water retention
- Lethargy and low stamina
- Weak immune system
- TMJ tension and pain
- Unruly appetite

Emotional Issues
- Anxiety, excessive worry
- Lack of focus or awareness
- Overprotective behaviors
- Obsessive behaviors

Location and Flow of the Spleen Meridian

The Spleen meridian begins on the caudomedial aspect of the coronary band of the hind leg, about two-thirds of the way toward the bulb of the heel from the midline. It proceeds up the medial aspect of the hind leg over the pastern, and metatarsus, turns slightly cranial and passes over the medial aspect of the hock, up the medial aspect of the back of the tibia, crosses the stifle and continues to a point in front of the tuber coxae. The meridian continues toward the head, traveling along the ventral abdomen and chest to the fourth intercostal space, at the level of the elbow. The Spleen meridian then turns and travels caudally, ending in the tenth intercostal space, approximately level with the point of the shoulder where Spleen 21, the last acupoint on the meridian, is found.

SPLEEN MERIDIAN

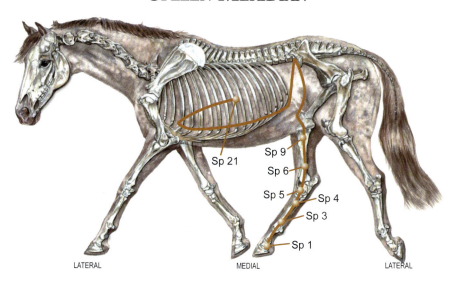

Point	Energetics/Function	Location
Sp 1	Jing-Well point. Regulates the Spleen, facilitates blood flow, contains the blood, calms the spirit and clears the brain. **Benefits** abdominal pain or distension, lack of appetite, uterine bleeding, convulsions, and shock. Benefits laminitis.	On the caudomedial aspect of the hind hoof proximal to the the coronary band.
Sp 3	Source point. Regulates and strengthens the Spleen, regulates the Stomach and Large Intestine, clears Heat, reduces digestive stagnation. **Benefits** the spine, ringbone, or hock arthritis.	Found on the distal end of the medial splint bone.
Sp 4	Connecting point. Regulates and strengthens the Spleen, chi and Yang. Regulates the Stomach, and relieves digestive stagnation. **Benefits** the Stomach, colic, abdominal, distension, suppressed appetite, and chronic diarrhea.	Located in a depression on the hind leg, mediodistal to the head of the medial splint bone.

Spleen Meridian

Point	Energetics/Function	Location
Sp 5	Regulates and strengthens the Spleen, transforms Damp-Heat. **Benefits** abdominal and hock pain, diarrhea and constipation.	On the saphenous vein, in a depression cranial and distal to the medial malleolus.
Sp 6	Master point for the urogenital system and the rear portion of the abdomen. Regulates, strengthens, and tonifies the Spleen. Regulates the Stomach, reduces digestive stagnation, tonifies chi and blood, nourishes blood. Tonifies the Kidneys enriches Yin, and promotes urination. Regulates estrous, invigorates the blood, and cools Heat in the blood. Regulates the Liver. Softens hard masses. **Benefits** hyperthyroidism, edema, spontaneous sweating, fatigued extremities, or chronic loose manure. Use for dry skin or urinary tract infection. Benefits impotence or sterility, urinary incontinence or retention, irregular estrous, lower back pain, and stifle pain. Benefits difficult labor or retained placenta, paralysis or motor impairment, or pain on the medial aspect of the stifle. Strengthens the immune system. Contraindicated during pregnancy	Found 3 cun above the tip of the medial malleolus, caudal to the tibial border, on the medial aspect of hind leg. 0.5 cun posterior to the saphenous vein of the hindlimb.
Sp 9	Regulates and strengthens the Spleen, regulates Stomach and water pathways. **Benefits** Yin deficiency conditions, edema, urinary incontinence, stifle pain, and arthritis.	In depression at the level of the patellar ligaments, 0.5 cun in front of the saphenous vein.
Sp 21	Connecting point of all Connecting points. Expands and relaxes the chest, regulates chi and blood, tonifies Nutritive chi, and facilitates chi and blood flow throughout the body. Controls all Yin meridians. **Benefits** all types of blood diseases, generalized body pain, fatigue, heaves, and general weakness. Fills in gaps in chi in the body and benefits flaccid and weak joints.	At the level of the shoulder joint in the 10th intercostal space.

HEART
Foreleg *Shaoyin* / Lesser Yin
Home of the *Shen* / Spirit

The Heart is known as the "Monarch" or "Ruler" of the entire body because of its important role in blood circulation. Heart chi must be vigorous to nourish the horse's body. Mental consciousness and the *shen*/spirit of the animal is said to reside in the Heart.

In Chinese thought, "consciousness" has a broad meaning and refers to the overall appearance and self-presentation of the horse. Consciousness is the vitality of the animal. When a horse is content and healthy, he will "strut his stuff." When a horse is not well or upset, you will know it immediately by his demeanor. The spirit, or *shen*, of the animal is said to be "Housed in the Heart and revealed in the eyes." Known in Chinese as *Xin*, the Heart is the yin organ system paired with the Small Intestine yang organ system.

Functions and Attributes
- Governs the direction and strength of blood flow and pulse
- Controls the blood vessels
- Regulates the nervous system
- Houses the mind and shen /spirit
- Regulates body heat
- Sensory orifice is the tongue
- Fluid is sweat
- Emotion is joy
- Belongs to the Fire Element
- Optimal flow of chi 11 AM–1 PM

Health Issues
- Cardiovascular disorders
- Shoulder pain
- Atrophy, tension or swelling of the neck
- Brain or nervous system disorders
- Spontaneous or excessive sweating
- Swollen or abnormal color of tongue

Emotional Issues
- Lack of joy /depression
- Lack of mental clarity or focus
- Mania /shen disturbance
- Restlessness and anxiety
- Nervous exhaustion

Location and Flow of the Heart Meridian

The Heart meridian begins close to the heart in the axilla area (armpit). It travels down the foreleg on the caudomedial side of the ulna toward the carpus. Here it crosses laterally over the carpus and continues down the caudolateral aspect of the foreleg. The Heart meridian ends at a point one-third of the distance from the heel bulb to the midpoint of the hoof. This is the Jing-Well point, Heart 9.

Heart Meridian

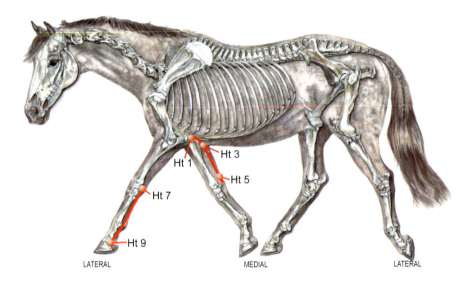

Point	Energetics/Function	Location
Ht 1	Regulates the Heart, facilitates chi flow. **Benefits** shoulder lameness, Yin deficiency, and shen disturbances.	At the center of the axilla, between the trunk and forelimb.
Ht 3	Regulates the Heart, chi and blood. Calms the spirit and strengthens the brain. **Benefits** elbow and thoracic pain. Seizures or shen disturbances.	Found between the olecranon crease and the medial epicondyle of the humerus.
Ht 5	Connecting point. Regulates and tonifies the Heart, Heart chi and Yang. Calms the spirit and strengthens the brain. **Benefits** anxiety, restlessness, and carpal pain.	Found on the caudal aspect of the radius, in a depression at about the level of the accessory carpal bone.

Heart Meridian

Point	Energetics/Function	Location
Ht 7	Source point. Regulates and tonifies the Heart and clears Heat. Calms the spirit, strengthens and clears the brain. **Benefits** mania, seizures, depression, hyperactivity, anxiety and fright, arthritis of the carpal joint, and is a reflex point for the shoulder, fetlock, and hoof.	Found on the caudolateral aspect of the radius proximal to the accessory carpal bone. Opposite Pe 7.
Ht 9	Jing-Well point. Regulates the Heart, redirects rebellious chi downward, revives consciousness, and clears the brain. **Benefits** chest pain, fever, sudden loss of consciousness, shen disturbances, and thoracic or shoulder lameness, and laminitis.	Found on the caudolateral aspect of the front hoof proximal to the coronary band.

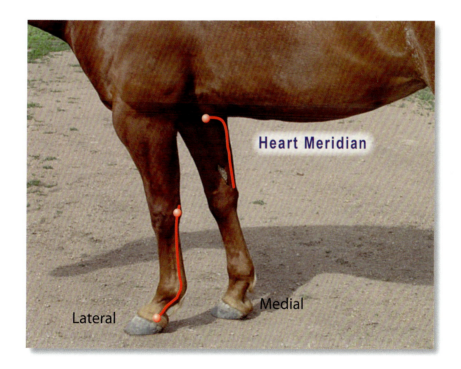

SMALL INTESTINE
Foreleg *Taiyang* /Greater Yang
Controller of Assimilation

The Small Intestine plays an important part in digestion. It receives the remains of the fluids and food not absorbed by the initial digestive process in the Stomach and Spleen. The Small Intestine is responsible for separating the clean from the turbid and absorbing the clean, usable fluids and nutrients. Hence, the Small Intestine, called *Xiao Chang* in Chinese, is instrumental in the assimilation of nutrients.

The Small Intestine's role of separating pure from impure has further implications. The Small Intestine provides the capacity to discern right from wrong and the ability to distinguish relevant issues with clarity. The Small Intestine is the yang organ system paired with the Heart. It keeps the Monarch's kingdom of the body pure and offers clarity of mind to make fair, diplomatic judgments.

Functions and Attributes
- Controls receiving and transforming
- Separates clean from turbid
- Provides the power of discernment
- Regulates the function of the intestines
- Regulates the absorption of body fluids
- Belongs to the Fire Element
- Optimal flow of chi 1–3 PM

Health Issues
- Arm, shoulder, and neck pain
- Atrophy, tension or swelling of the neck
- Digestion or absorption problems
- TMJ tension or pain
- Dental problems
- Urinary and bowel problems

Emotional Issues
- Not knowing right from wrong
- Lack of joy /depression
- Lack of mental clarity or confusion
- Manic behavior /shen disturbance
- Restlessness and anxiety

Location and Flow of the Small Intestine Meridian

The Small Intestine meridian begins on the craniolateral aspect of the coronary band at a point about one-third the distance from the front to the rear of the hoof. Staying on the craniolateral side of the forelimb, it travels up, over the pastern and cannon bone, over the carpus, and upper leg. It flows over the triceps muscle and scapula moving cranially along the neck. It touches the jaw bone and ends at a point on the lateral side of the ear base. The Small Intestine meridian has 19 acupoints along its pathway.

Small Intestine Meridian

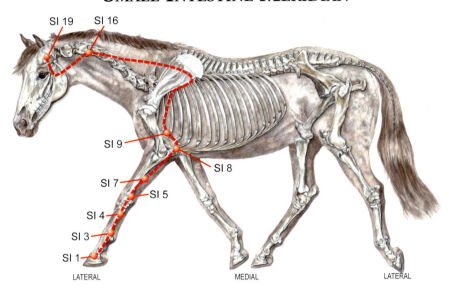

Point	Energetics/Function	Location
SI 1	Jing-Well point. Clears Heat and moistens Dryness, revives consciousness, and opens the sensory orifices. **Benefits** insufficient lactation, fever, coma, laminitis, or shoulder pain.	Located on the craniolateral aspect of the front hoof proximal to the coronary band.
SI 3	Stimulates sweating, regulates the Governing Vessel, relaxes sinews and alleviates pain. **Benefits** the fetlock, tendinitis, stiffness and neck pain, shoulder and back pain, laminitis, seizures, and mania.	In a depression on the distal end of the lateral splint bone on the caudolateral border of the cannon bone.
SI 4	Source point. Relaxes the sinews, dispels Wind-Heat, and transforms Damp-Heat. **Benefits** arthritis of the carpal and fetlock joints, tendinitis, and neck stiffness.	Found on the lateral surface of the forelimb at the level of the lateral splint bone.
SI 5	Clears Heat, opens sensory orifices, calms the spirit. **Benefits** hoof and shoulder issues, all disorders of the carpal joint.	In a depression on the lateral epicondyle of radius, cranial to Ht 7.
SI 7	Connecting point. Dispels Wind, clears Heat and stimulates sweating. **Benefits** elbow and forelimb pain, and neck stiffness or pain.	On the caudolateral aspect of the forelimb, about 6 cun above SI 5.

Small Intestine Meridian

Point	Energetics/Function	Location
SI 8	Dispels Wind and relaxes the sinews. **Benefits** elbow, neck and shoulder pain, and seizures.	Located in a depression between the elbow and the lateral epicondyle of the humerus.
SI 9	Dispels Wind. **Benefits** shoulder and neck pain, forelimb lameness, reduces inflammation and general pain.	In a depression at the caudal border of the deltoid muscle where it meets the lateral and long heads of the triceps brachii.
SI 16	Regulates chi, calms the spirit & clears Heat. **Benefits** neck stiffness and pain, reflex point for ligament or tendon issues.	At the level of the 2nd cervical vertebral space, dorsal border of the brachiocephalicus muscle.
SI 19	Clears Heat, opens the ears & calms spirit. **Benefits** auditory dysfunction, mania or anxiety.	Located in a depression at the rostral (toward the front of head) lateral corner of the ear base.

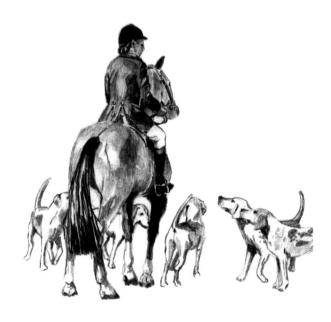

BLADDER
Hind Leg *Taiyang*/Greater Yang
Great Mediator

The Bladder is responsible for storing and excreting urine as well as producing chi transformation of fluids to moisten the Lung. This yang organ system is paired with the Kidney and dominated by the Kidney. In Chinese the Bladder is known as *Pang Guang*.

Unlike the other 12 Major Meridians, the Bladder meridian has two superficial branches with acupoints that flow on the dorsal aspect of the horse's back. The most medial branch, or channel, has a unique classification of acupoints called the Association points, or Back *Shu* points. These acupoints are directly connected to each of the 12 yin and yang internal organs. For instance, Bladder 13 is the Lung Association point and Bladder 15 is the Heart Association point. Because each of these acupoints is connected to an organ, you can use these points for both assessment and point work during the acupressure session.

Functions and Attributes
- Stores fluids and excretes urine
- Removes fluid by chi transformation
- Belongs to the Water Element
- Optimal flow of chi 3–5 PM

Health Issues
- Urinary tract problems
- Back and lower back soreness
- Dry lungs
- Low physical energy
- Body fluid problems

Emotional Issues
- Excessive or chronic anxiety
- Fear issues
- Jealousy

Location and Flow of the Bladder Meridian

The Bladder meridian begins at the inner corner of the horse's eye, traveling over the head and passing the wings of the atlas. It flows down the neck and over the withers, where it splits into two branches. The two branches follow lines parallel to the spine. The top channel runs 3 cun off the spine, the second channel runs 6 cun lateral to the dorsal midline. The channels flow down the back toward the tail, merging around Bl 40. The channel continues down the caudolateral aspect of the hind leg and ends at Bl 67, the Jing-Well point. This point is at the coronary band, about two-thirds of the distance from the front to the back of the hoof.

BLADDER MERIDIAN

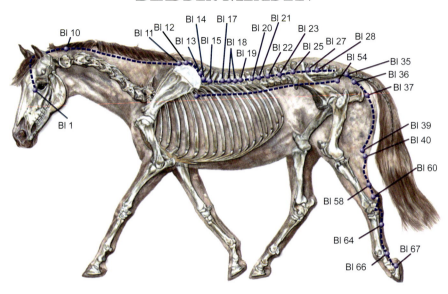

Point	Energetics/Function	Location
Bl 1	Opens and brightens the eyes, dispels Wind, and enriches Yin. **Benefits** all eye disorders including uveitis, conjunctivitis, and optic nerve atrophy.	In the indentation at the medial canthus of the eye.
Bl 10	Opens sensory orifices, dispels Wind and Cold and clears Heat. **Benefits** the eyes, nasal congestion, and neck stiffness.	Two cun off the dorsal midline in a depression caudal to the wings of the atlas.
Bl 11	Influential point for Bone and Sea of Blood point. Relaxes sinews, strengthens bone and joints. Nourishes and facilitates blood flow. **Benefits** osteoarthritis, joint problems or deformities, neck and spinal pain and stiffness, cough or fever. Tonic for internal conditions.	One and one-half cun lateral to dorsal midline at about the 3rd thoracic vertebra, cranial to the withers.
Bl 12	Influential point for Wind and Trachea. Regulates the Lung, dispels Wind, and strengthens Protective chi. **Benefits** cervical and thoracic pain, nasal congestion, cough, itchy skin, and fever.	Found at the highest point of the withers at about the 4th thoracic vertebral space.

BLADDER MERIDIAN

Point	Energetics/Function	Location
BL 13	Association point for Lung. Regulates and tonifies the Lung, diffuses Lung chi. **Benefits** any respiratory condition, stimulates sweating, neck or back stiffness, atrophy syndrome.	Three cun lateral to the dorsal midline in the 8th intercostal space.
Bl 14	Association point for the Pericardium. Regulates and tonifies the Heart, helps spread Liver chi. **Benefits** anxiety and palpitations, cough, heart irregularities or disease.	Three cun lateral to the dorsal midline in the 9th intercostal space.
Bl 15	Association point for the Heart. Regulates and tonifies the Heart, calms the spirit, and clears the brain. **Benefits** cardiac pain or palpitations, anxiety, seizures or disorientation.	Three cun lateral to the dorsal midline in the 10th intercostal space.
Bl 17	Influential point for Blood and the Diaphragm. Regulates and tonifies the Spleen, regulates and tonifies the blood, and enriches Yin. **Benefits** low hemoglobin count, blood pressure, wasting diseases, fatigue, nonresponsive skin conditions, immunostimulation.	Three cun lateral to the dorsal midline in the 12th intercostal space.
Bl 18	Association point for Liver. Regulates and tonifies the Liver, regulates GB, facilitates chi flow and brightens the eyes, and softens hard masses. **Benefits** seizures, muscular tetany, atrophy, jaundice or hepatitis, or abdominal pain. Benefits chronic fatigue.	Three cun lateral to the dorsal midline in the 13th and 14th intercostal spaces.
Bl 19	Association point for Gall Bladder. Regulates the Liver and GB, clears Liver Heat, expels parasites, softens hard masses. **Benefits** eye disorders, pain in the hip, sciatica, myositis, tendinitis or gastrointestinal problems. Work this point after giving your horse a natural de-wormer.	Three cun lateral to the dorsal midline in the 15th intercostal space.

BLADDER MERIDIAN

Point	Energetics/Function	Location
BL 20	Association point for Spleen. Regulates and tonifies the Spleen, tonifies Nutritive chi and blood, reduces digestive stagnation. **Benefits** edema, diarrhea, anemia, and gastrointestinal disorders.	Three cun lateral to the dorsal midline in the last (17th) intercostal space.
Bl 21	Association point for Stomach. Regulates the Stomach and tonifies the Spleen. **Benefits** atrophy syndrome, gastrointestinal disorders, edema, back pain and general weakness.	Three cun lateral to the dorsal midline caudal to the last rib.
Bl 22	Association point for Triple Heater. Regulates the Triple Heater, tonifies the Kidneys and resolves dampness. **Benefits** hormonal imbalances, edema, chronic nephritis, and urinary issues.	Three cun lateral to the dorsal midline between the 1st and 2nd lumbar vertebrae.
Bl 23	Association point for Kidney. Tonifies Kidney Essence, warms Yang, and tonifies Source chi. **Benefits** general weakness, seizures, ears and eyes, lower back pain, the brain, estrous cycles, and impotence.	Three cun lateral to the dorsal midline between the 2nd and 3rd lumbar vertebrae, directly dorsal to the ventral end of the last rib.
Bl 25	Association point for Large Intestine. Regulates the LI and warms Cold. **Benefits** all intestinal disorders, constipation or diarrhea, back pain or stiffness. Strengthens the lower back.	Three cun lateral to the dorsal midline between the 5th and 6th lumbar vertebrae at the cranial edge of the wings of the ilium.
Bl 27	Association point for Small Intestine. Regulates the Small Intestine and stabilizes Essence. **Benefits** caudal abdominal pain, colic, and lower back pain.	Three cun lateral to the dorsal midline between the 1st and 2nd sacral vertebrae.
Bl 28	Association point for Bladder. Regulates the Bladder, water pathways, and clears Heat. **Benefits** urinary dysfunction, constipation and diarrhea, and abdominal pain and distension.	Three cun lateral to the dorsal midline between the 2nd and 3rd sacral vertebrae.
Bl 35	Clears Heat. **Benefits** tail paralysis, and diarrhea. Is a reflex point for the hock.	Found in the muscle groove 2 cun craniolateral to the root of the tail.

BLADDER MERIDIAN

Point	Energetics/Function	Location
Bl 36	Facilitates chi flow. **Benefits** the lower back, gluteal pain, and inflammation.	Found in the muscle groove at the level of the center of the anus.
Bl 37	Activates the channel and alleviates pain. **Benefits** hind limb lameness, muscular atrophy, pelvic limb paralysis, and sciatica.	Found in the muscle groove at the level of the tuber ischii.
Bl 39	Regulates Triple Heater, Bladder, and water pathways. **Benefits** urinary issues, edema, hock issues. Reflex point for hock.	Found at the ventral edge of the muscle groove at the level of the stifle, cranial to Bl 40.
Bl 40	Master point for the back and hips. Dispels Wind, clears Heat and moves blood. **Benefits** lower back and hips, stifle disorders, gastrocnemius muscle spasms, sciatica, and urinary issues.	Located at the midpoint of the transverse crease of the popliteal fossa.
Bl 54	Strengthens the lower back. **Benefits** gluteal muscles, lower back and sacral pain, paralysis of hip and lower extremities. Helps immune-mediated issues.	Located just dorsal to the greater trochanter of the femur.
Bl 58	Connecting point. Dispels Wind. **Benefits** back pain, hock and hind limb pain.	Seven cun above Bl 60 on the caudal border of fibula.
Bl 60	Strengthens the lower back, relaxes the sinews, facilitates chi flow and blood, alleviates pain and swelling throughout body. **Benefits** arthritis of the hock, lumbar area and distal hind limb. Expedites labor. Contraindicated in pregnancy.	Found between the lateral malleolus of the tibia and the calcaneal tuber. Opposite Ki 3.
Bl 64	Source point. Calms the spirit clears Heat. **Benefits** cervical stiffness and back pain.	Located caudodistal to the head of the lateral splint bone.
Bl 66	Calms the spirit and clears Heat. **Benefits** navicular and arthritis of the fetlock.	Found distal to the fetlock on the caudolateral aspect of the pastern, hind leg.
Bl 67	Jing-Well point. Regulates chi and blood, clears Heat. **Benefits** laminitis, clears the nose and brightens the eyes, promotes parturition. Contraindicated in pregnancy.	On the caudolateral aspect of coronary band of the hind leg.

KIDNEY
Hind Leg *Shaoyin* /Lesser Yin
Residence of Resolution

The Kidney organ system is called the "Root of Life" because it stores the substantive foundation of the horse's life. The Kidney stores Original, or Source, chi. Kidney chi is the original yin and yang of the body that the foal inherits from the dam and the sire. It's the *Jing*, or essence, with which the foal arrives on earth. This essence becomes depleted over the years until none remains and death ensues. Essence chi determines the physical and emotional strength and constitutional vitality of the animal.

The relationship of the Kidney and the Lung is significant and forms the inner core strength of the body. Lung chi descends and Kidney chi must be strong enough to grasp and "root the breath." The animal's will power, *zhi*, reflects this core strength in his force of determination.

Kidney, *Shen* in Chinese, is the yin organ system paired with the Bladder, which is yang. Together they are heavily involved in the functioning of the body's water metabolism.

Functions and Attributes
- Stores Jing chi /Essence chi
- Governs birth, growth, reproduction, and development
- Produces marrow and fills the brain
- Controls bones and manufactures blood
- Dominates water metabolism
- Controls the reception and grasping of Lung chi
- Controls the lower two orifices
- Houses willpower
- Manifests in the quality of hair
- Sensory orifice is the ear
- Fluid is heavy phlegm (spittle)
- Emotion is fear
- Belongs to the Water Element
- Optimal flow of chi 5–7 PM

Health Issues
- Lower back and back pain
- Hock and stifle problems
- Bone and arthritis problems
- Lack of physical energy
- Urinary tract problems
- Reproductive, fertility, and estrous cycle problems
- Development issues
- Dental issues
- Loss of hearing
- Ear problems

Emotional Issues
- Excessive or chronic anxiety
- Fear issues
- Jealousy

Location and Flow of the Kidney Meridian

The Kidney meridian starts at the coronary band on the hind leg at a point between the heel bulbs, known as Ki 1. The meridian travels up the caudomedial aspect of the hind leg to the hock. It circles the hock and continues its flow up the medial aspect of the hind leg to the groin area. It flows cranially along the ventral abdomen about 1 cun off the ventral midline. At the ribcage it flows 2 cun off the midline, through the chest, ending at Ki 27. There are 27 acupoints along the Kidney meridian.

NOTE: The Kidney meridian actually ends on the bottom of the hoof, on the frog. For ease of access, the depression between the bulbs of the heel is used as the end point.

KIDNEY MERIDIAN

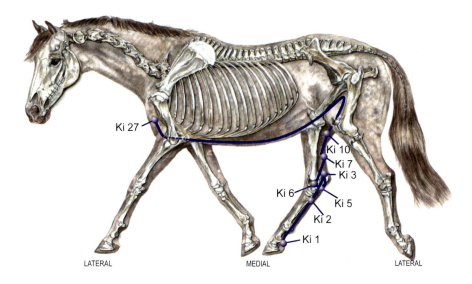

Point	Energetics/Function	Location
Ki 1	Jing-Well point. Tonifies the Kidneys and enriches Yin. Calms the spirit, restores consciousness. **Benefits** infertility, back or abdominal pain, constipation or diarrhea, laminitis, seizures, coma, heatstroke, and fever.	Located on the hind leg in the depression between the heel bulbs.
Ki 2	Clears Heat, regulates the Kidneys. **Benefits** abnormal cycling, impotence, infertility, spontaneous sweating and throat issues.	Found proximal to the medial splint bone in a depression below the 1st and 2nd tarsal bones.

Kidney Meridian

Point	Energetics/Function	Location
Ki 3	Source point. Tonifies the Kidneys, Source chi, blood, and essence. Restores collapsed Yin, calms the fetus, strengthens the brain, regulates estrous cycles, and water metabolism. **Benefits** arthritis and swelling of the hock, lower back pain, paralysis of the pelvic limb, kidney dysfunction, parturition, estrous cycle irregularity, and urinary incontinence or retention.	Located in the depression between the medial malleolus of the tibia and the calcaneal tuber. Opposite Bl 60.
Ki 5	Tonifies the Kidneys and regulates the Bladder. **Benefits** irregular cycling, anestrous, and painful urination	One cun below Ki 3, caudal to the distal end of the tibia.
Ki 6	Nourishes the Kidneys and clears deficiency Heat. **Benefits** eye pain, dysuria, abnormal cycling, constipation, and seizures.	Found in a depression between the calcaneal tuber and the talus.
Ki 7	Tonifies Kidney Yang, relieves dampness, regulates sweating. **Benefits** edema, abdomnal fullness, non-sweating.	Found about 2 cun above Ki 3 on the cranial border of the Achilles tendon.
Ki 10	Tonifies Kidney Yin, activates the channel and alleviates pain. **Benefits** impotence, stifle pain, dysuria or lower abdominal pain.	Found on the medial side of the popliteal fossa at the level of Bl 40, between the semimembranosus and semitendinosus muscles.
Ki 27	Association point of all Association points. Regulates the Lungs, tonfies Ancestral chi, and directs rebellious chi downward. **Benefits** mental fatigue, anxiety, lack of appetite, heaves, chest pain, and cough.	Located between the sternum and the 1st rib, 2 cun lateral to the ventral midline.

PERICARDIUM
Foreleg *Jueyin* /Absolute Yin
Heart Protector

The Pericardium, *Xin Bao* in Chinese, is the sheathing surrounding the heart. Because the Heart is the Monarch of the body, the Pericardium's role is to protect the Heart from physical and emotional insult. As the Heart Protector, the Pericardium is an active agent of the Heart by assisting the Heart in all of its functions. Additionally, the Pericardium is often used as a surrogate for the Heart. In fact, the Heart cannot be sedated directly, but the Pericardium can be sedated instead when needed.

Many Chinese texts don't consider the Pericardium an organ system but rather an appendage to the Heart. However, the yin Pericardium meridian and its associated acupoints are as powerful and commonly used as any of the 12 Major Meridians. The Pericardium is paired with the yang Triple Heater organ system.

Functions and Attributes
- Protects the Heart from external or internal pathogens
- Assists the Heart in cardiovascular functions
- Assists in balancing emotions
- Emotion is trust /intimacy
- Belongs to the Fire Element
- Optimal flow of chi 7–9 PM

Health Issues
- Chest pain or tension
- Forelimb pain or soreness
- Cardiovascular problems
- Blood stasis or deficiency

Emotional Issues
- Bonding difficulty
- Lack of trust
- Lack of mental clarity
- Timidity
- Abandonment issues
- Anxiety

Location and Flow of the Pericardium Meridian

The Pericardium meridian begins deep within the body at the sac that surrounds the heart. The meridian surfaces in the space between the 5th and 6th ribs, near the elbow. From here, it travels down the medial aspect of the foreleg in front of the chestnut. The meridian continues its flow down the caudomedial aspect of the leg, past the accessory carpal bone to Pe 9, a point between the bulbs of the heel.

Pericardium Meridian

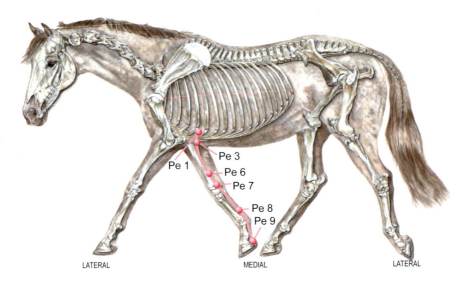

Point	Energetics/Function	Location
Pe 1	Regulates chi, clears Heat, and expands the chest. **Benefits** cough, insufficient lactation, and chest pain. Reflex point for front hoof.	Located in the 5th intercostal space medial to the point of the elbow.
Pe 3	Regulates Heart, Stomach and intestines. **Benefits** heatstroke, shoulder or elbow pain and fever.	Found on the medial side of the cubital crease of the elbow, cranial to Heart 3.
Pe 6	Connecting point. Master point for chest and cranial abdomen. Regulates and tonifies the Heart, facilitates chi flow, regulates the Yin-linking vessel. Calms the spirit and clears the brain. Expedites and facilitates lactation, and redirects rebellious chi downward. **Benefits** seizures, and severe agitation. Helps with asthma, contracture or pain in the elbow and foreleg.	Located on the medial aspect of the foreleg, about 2 cun above Pe 7, directly cranial to the mid-level of the chestnut.

Pericardium Meridian

Point	Energetics/Function	Location
Pe 7	Source point. Harmonizes the stomach and intestines, regulates the Heart, calms the spirit. **Benefits** epilepsy, stomach issues, and anxiety. Local point for the carpus.	Located at the level of the accessory carpal bone on the medial aspect of the foreleg.
Pe 8	Regulates the Heart, revives consciousness, and clears the brain. **Benefits** febrile issues, ulcers of the mouth, and shen disturbances.	Halfway between the carpus and the fetlock on the caudal aspect of the superficial digital flexor tendon.
Pe 9	Jing-Well point. Regulates the Heart, revives consciousness, restores collapsed Yang. **Benefits** sweating, laminitis, heatstroke, shock, and hyperactivity.	At the center of the depression between the heel bulbs on the forelimb.

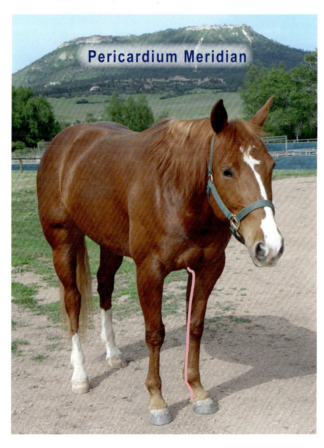

Triple Heater
Foreleg *Shaoyang* / Lesser Yang
Commander of All Energies

The Triple Heater, known in Chinese as *San Jiao,* is an esoteric aspect of Chinese medicine. It's viewed as an energetic organ and a functional system. As an energetic organ, it doesn't have a tangible form.

The Triple Heater is responsible for transforming and transporting chi so it flows unimpeded to all parts of the body. In this role, it assists in transforming and transporting nourishment and excreting waste as well as directing chi to all the organs. As an organ, it's the largest of the body, dividing the trunk into three distinct compartments—"heaters" or "burners." The upper heater includes the Lung, Heart, and Pericardium. The middle heater includes the Spleen and Stomach. The lower heater includes the Large and Small Intestine, Gall Bladder, Liver, Kidney, and Bladder. The Triple Heater is responsible for ensuring that all of the organs work in concert with each other.

The Triple Heater is called the "Avenue of Original Chi" because of its role in transporting Original chi to the 12 Major Meridians. The Original chi resides in the Kidney and is transported by the Triple Heater to surface at the Source points on each meridian. The Triple Heater is also involved in the function of the body's endocrine and lymphatic systems. The Pericardium is the yin meridian paired with the Triple Heater yang meridian.

Functions and Attributes

- Directs Original chi to the organs and Source points
- Coordinates the three energetic compartments
- Responsible for thermoregulation
- Regulates water passages
- Belongs to the Fire Element
- Optimal flow of chi 9–11 PM

Health Issues

- Forelimb, neck, and head pain, stiffness, or soreness
- Immune system issues (lymphatic system)
- Hormonal imbalance
- Temporomandibular (TMJ) issues
- Ear problems / deafness
- Eye issues
- Poor temperature regulation
- Climate sensitivity
- Metabolic problems
- Edema

Emotional Issues

- Depression
- Nervous anxiety

Location and Flow of the Triple Heater Meridian

The Triple Heater meridian starts at the midpoint of the coronary band on the forelimb. It flows up the cranial aspect of the pastern and cannon bone to the carpus. It continues up the lateral side of the foreleg past the elbow along the top side of the humerus to the caudal edge of the shoulder joint (TH 14). From here, it crosses the lower scapula and continues up the neck, around the ear, and ends at the supraorbital ridge above the eye. The Triple Heater meridian has 23 acupoints along its pathway.

TRIPLE HEATER MERIDIAN

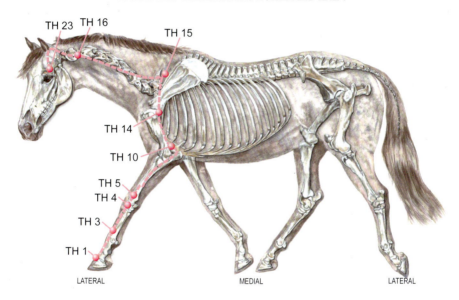

Point	Energetics/Function	Location
TH 1	Jing-Well point. Dispels Wind, revives consciousness, opens the sensory orifices. **Benefits** laminitis, fever, conjunctivitis, auditory dysfunction, colic, or shoulder pain.	Found just lateral to the cranial midline of the front hoof, proximal to the coronary band.
TH 3	Clears heat and dispels Wind. **Benefits** ear and eye disorders, pastern or fetlock pain, febrile issues or head shaking.	Found just lateral to the cranial midline of the fetlock 1/3rd up the cannon bone.
TH 4	Source point. Dispels Wind, clears Fire and Heat, relaxes the sinews, and alleviates pain. **Benefits** swelling, arthritis and sprain of the carpal joint, edema of the front leg, and relieves shoulder and foreleg pain.	Found in the large depression slightly lateral to the middle of the cranial surface of the carpal joint, between the intermediate and 3rd carpal bones.

Triple Heater Meridian

Point	Energetics/Function	Location
TH 5	Connecting point. Regulates the Triple Heater, clears Heat and tonifies Protective chi. **Benefits** febrile issues, strengthens the sinews, and alleviates pain.	Found between the radius and ulna 2 cun above TH 4. Opposite Pe 6.
TH 10	Dispels Wind, clears Heat, and calms spirit. **Benefits** paralysis of forelimbs, auditory issues, cervical and dental pain.	Found in a depression 1 cun craniodorsal to SI 8.
TH 14	Dispels Wind and Cold, relaxes the sinews. **Benefits** all shoulder conditions including inflammation, pain, and atrophy.	On the caudal edge of the shoulder joint at the level of the point of the shoulder.
TH 15	Regulates chi, activates the channel and alleviates pain. **Benefits** cervical stiffness, shoulder and front limb pain.	Located in a depression on the front border of the scapula.
TH 16	Regulates and descends chi. **Benefits** head shaking, auditory dysfunction, TMJ pain, Wobbler's Syndrome, and cervical stiffness.	Found between the 1st and 2nd cervical vertebrae, at the caudal border of the brachiocephalicus muscle.
TH 23	Brightens the eyes, clears Heat and dispels Wind. **Benefits** all eye disorders, facial paralysis, dental diseases, encephalitis, and epilepsy.	One cun above GB 1, near the lateral canthus of the eye, and caudal to the orbit.

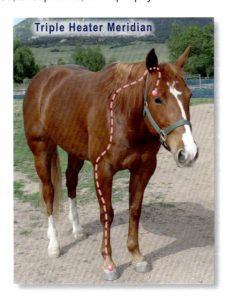

GALL BLADDER
Hind leg *Shaoyang* /Lesser Yang
Official of Decision-making and Judgment

The Gall Bladder stores and excretes bile as needed for digestion. This yang organ system is paired with the Liver, a yin organ system. The functions of the Gall Bladder are closely related to the Liver's capacity to provide a harmonious flow of chi. Known in Chinese as *Dan*, the Gall Bladder assists the Liver in many of its functions. This organ system is thought to affect the animal's courage and ability to take initiative and make decisions. Many physical issues can be addressed using the Gall Bladder meridian because it's one of the longest meridians in the body, extending from head to hind hoof.

Functions and Attributes
- Stores and excretes bile
- Governs decision-making/judgment
- Assists in Liver function
- Belongs to the Wood Element
- Optimal flow of chi 11PM–1AM
- Hoof problems
- Stiff or cramped muscles
- Vision or eye issues
- Neck, shoulder, hip, stifle, and hock problems
- Toxic issues

Health Issues
- Digestive disorders
- Muscle spasms, seizures, convulsions
- Tendon-related pain or disorders

Emotional Issues
- Depression
- Lack of initiative
- Indecisiveness
- Aggressiveness or anger

Location and Flow of the Gall Bladder Meridian

Gall Bladder 1 is located at the lateral canthus (corner) of the eye. It runs up toward the poll to the medial side of the ear, then flows cranially to a point above the eye and back to a point at a depression at the occipital condyle (GB 20). It then curves behind the ear and flows down the neck to the middle of the scapula and flows across the chest to the 14th intercostal space, GB 24. It travels up to GB 25, a point on the caudal border of the last rib. The meridian flows around the hip area and down the middle of the lateral aspect of the hind leg. GB 44, the last point on this meridian, is located at the craniolateral aspect of the coronary band, approximately one-third of the distance from the front to the back of the hoof. This is the Jing-Well point of the Gall Bladder meridian. There are 44 acupoints along the Gall Bladder meridian.

GALL BLADDER MERIDIAN

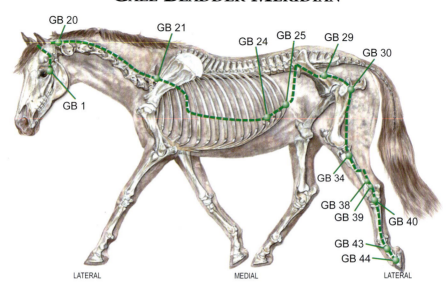

Point	Energetics/Function	Location
GB 1	Brightens the eyes, dispels Wind and clears Fire. **Benefits** ocular disorders, anhidrosis, and facial paralysis.	Located 1 cun caudoventral to the lateral canthus of the eye.
GB 20	Dispels Wind, subdues Liver-Yang, facilitates chi flow and clears the brain. **Benefits** cervical issues, seizures, and eye disorders.	Found in the large depression caudal to the occipital condyle.
GB 21	Spreads Liver chi, facilitates chi flow, and clears the brain. **Benefits** shoulder and neck pain, paralysis of forelimbs, expedites labor and facilitates lactation.	At the midpoint of the cranial edge of the scapula.
GB 24	Alarm point for GB. Regulates Liver, GB, and Stomach. Spreads Liver chi. **Benefits** fatigued extremities, liver issues, and moves stagnation.	Located at the 14th intercostal space, caudal and dorsal to Liv 14.
GB 25	Alarm point for Kidney. Tonifies the Kidneys, warms the Yang, and relaxes the sinews. Any Kidney imbalance is manifested as pain at this point. **Benefits** abdominal or lower back pain. Expels urinary tract stones.	Located at the caudal border of the last rib.

GALL BLADDER MERIDIAN

Point	Energetics/Function	Location
GB 29	Dispels Wind, Cold and clears Heat. **Benefits** lower back, hip joint disorders, gluteal muscle soreness, coxofemoral joint arthritis, and hind limb pain.	Located halfway between the wing of the ilium and the greater trochanter of the femur.
GB 30	Dispels Wind and Cold, clears Heat, and transforms dampness. **Benefits** lower back and hips, pelvic limb paresis or paralysis, and gluteal muscle pain.	Found on the caudoventral edge of the greater trochanter in a depression.
GB 34	Influential point for Tendons and Ligaments. Regulates and tonifies the Liver, regulates the Gall Bladder, spreads Liver chi, subdues Liver Yang, extinguishes Liver Wind, clears Heat, and drains Liver pathogens. **Benefits** atrophy and promotes the flow of blood and chi in the legs. Benefits weak tendons/ligaments, hind-end weakness and muscle cramps or spasms.	In the interosseous space between the tibia and fibula, between the long and lateral digital extensors, craniodistal to the head of the fibula.
GB 38	Clears Heat, activates the channel and relieves pain. **Benefits** eye problems, sinews and bones.	Found 1 cun above GB 39 between the lateral digital extensor and the deep digital flexor muscles.
GB 39	Influential point for Marrow. Clears GB Fire and dispels Wind-Damp. **Benefits** the sinews and bones, cervical issues, and paresis or paralysis of the hind limb.	Three cun above the tip of the lateral malleolus in a depression on the caudal aspect of the tibia.
GB 40	Source point. Regulates Liver and GB, and spreads Liver chi. **Benefits** pain in the distal extremities. Softens hard masses, and strengthens the hock.	Craniodistal to the tip of lateral malleolus of the tibia over the tendon of the lateral digital extensor.
GB 43	Clears Heat. **Benefits** the head, ears, and eyes. Helps laminitis, tendinitis, and hypertension.	Located on the lateral aspect of the hind limb distal to the fetlock joint.
GB 44	Jing-Well point. Clears the sensory orifices, calms the mind. **Benefits** laminits, arthritis, abnormal cycling, hock pain, and hip problems.	Found on the craniolateral aspect of the coronary band on the hind limb.

LIVER
Hind leg *Jueyin* /Absolute Yin
Controller of Strategic Planning

The Liver ensures the smooth, harmonious flow of chi throughout the horse's body. The Liver stores and replenishes blood while also managing the volume of blood in response to the demands of physical activity. Known as *Gan* in Chinese, the Liver plays a role in the energetics and nourishment of tissues for the entire body. It also plays a significant role in digestion.

As the Strategic Planner, the Liver is involved in all the body functions and the emotions; that is, all of the other internal organs are dependent on the proper functioning of the Liver. The Gallbladder is the yang organ system paired with the Liver.

Functions and Attributes
- Governs the harmonious flow of chi
- Stores and replenishes blood
- Regulates the volume of blood
- Controls the sinews (tendons and ligaments)
- Influences descending chi
- Manifests in hoof
- Sensory orifice is the eyes
- Fluid is bile
- Emotion is anger
- Belongs to the Wood Element
- Optimal flow of chi 1–3 AM

Health Issues
- Muscle spasms, seizures, convulsions
- Tendon and ligament problems
- Hoof issues
- Stiff or cramped muscles
- Vision or eye disorders
- Estrous cycle problems
- Reproductive issues
- Digestive problems
- Joint problems
- Toxic issues
- Low energy
- Blood disorders

Emotional Issues
- Depression
- Lack of initiative
- Aggressiveness or anger
- Erratic behavior
- Irritability

Location and Flow of the Liver Meridian

The Liver meridian begins on the hind leg at the craniomedial aspect of the coronary band at Liver 1. The meridian travels up the craniomedial aspect of the hind leg, over the pastern, cannon bone, and hock, shifting slightly forward as it travels up the tibia. It passes caudal to the medial condyle of the femur and enters the inguinal region. The meridian then turns and travels cranially. The next to the last point, Liver 13, is located at the end of the next to the last rib. Here the meridian slants down slightly and ends at Liver 14, located in the 13th intercostal space at the level of the elbow. There are 14 acupoints along the Liver meridian.

LIVER MERIDIAN

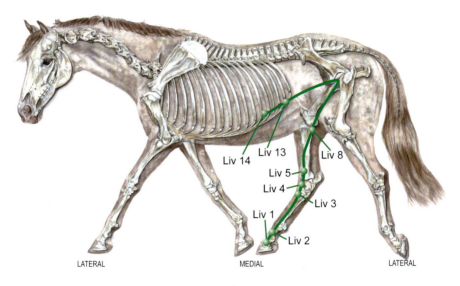

Point	Energetics/Function	Location
Liv 1	Jing-Well point. Regulates and tonifies the Liver, spreads Liver chi, and helps contain blood. **Benefits** laminitis and side bone, irregular estrous, hernia, or constipation.	Found on the craniomedial aspect of the hind hoof proximal to the coronary band.
Liv 2	Regulates Liver, invigorates blood, and calms the spirit. **Benefits** ocular disorders, laminitis, ringbone, and abnormal cycling.	Found on the medial aspect of the hind limb below the fetlock joint.
Liv 3	Source point. Regulates and tonifies the Liver, invigorates the blood, regulates chi. **Benefits** Liver and GB disorders, endocrine and metabolic disorders, eye issues, fetlock and hock pain, and toxin removal.	On the craniodistal aspect of the cannon bone at the level of the head of the medial splint bone.
Liv 4	Spreads Liver chi and regulates the lower Heater. **Benefits** hock pain and anhidrosis.	One cun in front of medial malleolus in a depression near the saphenous vein.
Liv 5	Connecting point. Regulates and tonifies Liver, spreads Liver chi and enriches Yin. **Benefits** impotence, irregular estrous, sterility, and muscle spasms of the back.	Located 2 cun proximal to Sp 6 on the cranial border of the tibia.

Liver Meridian

Point	Energetics/Function	Location
Liv 8	Nourishes blood and Yin. **Benefits** reproductive disorders, stifle pain, urinary incontinence, and abnormal cycling.	Found behind the medial condyle of the femur, in front of the tendons of the semimembranosus and semitendinosus.
Liv 13	Alarm point for Spleen, Influential point of Yin organs. Regulates, tonifies, and strengthens the Spleen, reduces digestive stagnation, and regulates the Stomach. **Benefits** food stagnation, abdominal masses and pain, and fatigued or painful extremities.	Found on the lateral side of abdomen on the lower margin of the 2nd to the last rib.
Liv 14	Alarm point for Liver. Regulates Liver and GB, spreads Liver chi, expands and relaxes the chest. **Benefits** the Liver and Stomach, stabilizes the emotions, lactation, and muscle pain.	Found at the 13th intercostal space at the level of the elbow.

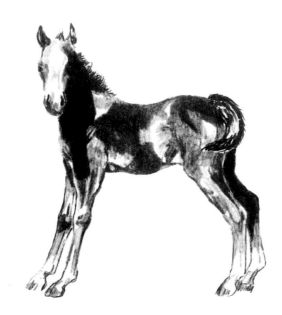

EXTRAORDINARY VESSELS

CONCEPTION VESSEL   GOVERNING VESSEL
Ren Mai   &   *Du Mai*
Yin Gathering Vessel   *Yang Gathering Vessel*

Eight Extraordinary Vessels, or channels, serve as storage, or reservoirs, for chi. Of the eight Extraordinary Vessels, two vessels—the Conception and Governing Vessels—are usually included with the 12 Major Meridians because they have their own acupoints. Although these two channels are not associated with a particular *zang-fu* organ, nor are they paired with each other, they are instrumental in maintaining the constant dynamic balance of yin and yang chi in the body. The remaining six Extraordinary Vessels don't have their own acupoints and the chi of those six vessels is accessed through points on the 12 Major Meridians.

The Conception Vessel, also known as the *Sea of Yin*, acts as a reservoir for yin chi. The other *zang-fu* organ systems can use the yin chi as needed to balance yang chi. Likewise, the Governing Vessel, also called the *Sea of Yang*, is the reservoir of yang chi and serves to balance the yin chi. The Conception Vessel and Governing Vessel are connected to create the continuous flow of yin and yang.

These two vessels receive energy from the Kidney and share the essence that's stored in the Kidney. Like all the Extraordinary Vessels, these vessels circulate Nutrient / *Ying* chi and Original chi and serve as the connection with the 12 Major Meridians. The Extraordinary Vessels function at a deeper level than the main channels and profoundly affect the constitution of the horse.

Conception Vessel
Ren Mai
Yin Gathering Vessel

The Conception Vessel absorbs, stores, and transfers yin chi as needed to maintain a dynamic balance within the 12 Major Meridians. The acupoints along this channel have a strong influence on the reproductive system, physical development, and the transportation of chi and blood to the lower compartment of the Triple Heater and uterus in the female. Additionally, these acupoints can be used to resolve organ issues along the horse's ventral midline. For instance, Conception Vessel 3, *Middle Extremity*, is located near the Bladder and is known to benefit urinary problems and enhance the Bladder's capacity to perform chi transformation.

Functions and Attributes
- Unites and balances the 12 Major Meridians
- Nourishes yin chi
- Governs reproduction and fertility
- Governs growth and development
- Governs the peripheral nervous system (outside the spinal column)
- Regulates blood flow in the 12 Major Meridians
- Replenishes Original chi

Health Issues
- Reproductivew/fertility issues
- Collapse of yang
- Blood problems
- Digestive issues
- Local pain/disorders

Emotional Issues
- Hyperactivity
- Anxiety

Location and Flow of the Conception Vessel

The Conception Vessel, called *Du Mai* in Chinese, travels the full length of the ventral midline on the horse's body. The meridian begins at a point below the anus (CV 1). It then runs between the hind legs, through the genitals and umbilicus, continuing along the ventral midline of the abdomen and through the chest. It continues cranially along the midline of the neck and head and ends at a point on the lower lip, Conception Vessel 24.

NOTE: This meridian runs only on the ventral midline of the horse and does not have a sister meridian.

Conception Vessel Meridian

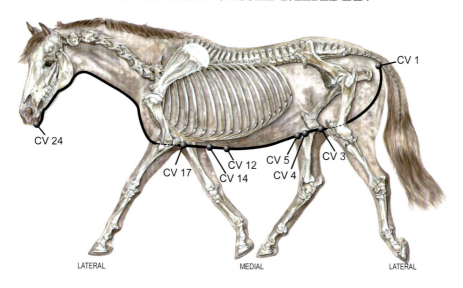

Point	Energetics/Function	Location
CV 1	Stabilizes the essence, tonifies and regulates chi, and revives consciousness. **Benefits** infertility, uterine prolapse, and seizures.	Located on the ventral midline halfway between the anus and the scrotum or vulva.
CV 3	Alarm point for Bladder. Regulates the lower Heater, clears Heat, and tonifies the Kidneys. **Benefits** infertility, impotence, incontinence, and dysuria.	Found on the ventral midline 4 cun caudal to the umbilicus.
CV 4	Alarm point for Small Intestine. Tonifies the Kidneys and Source chi, warms cold and enriches Yin. **Benefits** infertility, colic, organ prolapse, generalized weakness, coma, or shock. Benefits chronic consumptive disorders.	Found on the ventral midline 3 cun caudal to the umbilicus.
CV 5	Alarm point for the Triple Heater. Tonifies the Kidneys, Source chi, and warms Yang. **Benefits** abdominal pain, diarrhea, infertility, irregular estrous cycles, and general weakness.	Found on the ventral midline 2 cun caudal to the umbilicus.

Conception Vessel Meridian

Point	Energetics/Function	Location
CV 12	Alarm point for the Stomach. Influential point of the Yang organs. Regulates, strengthens and tonifies the Spleen, Stomach and middle Heater, tonifies Nutritive chi. **Benefits** anxiety or fear, cardiac arrhythmias, and gastrointestinal issues.	Found on the ventral midline halfway between the xiphoid process and the umbilicus.
CV 14	Alarm point for the Heart. Regulates the Heart and chi, calms the spirit. **Benefits** seizures, facial paralysis, upper body edema, and conjunctivitis.	Found on the ventral midline at about the level of the xiphoid process.
CV 17	Alarm point for the Pericardium. Influential point for the respiratory system and chi. Regulates the Lung, and regulates and tonifies the chi. **Benefits** all respiratory conditions, anxiety, breast disorders, and insufficient lactation.	Found on the ventral midline at the level of the caudal border of the elbow.
CV 24	Dispels Wind, and clears Heat. **Benefits** facial paralysis, behavioral issues, mania, seizures, and gum or tooth pain.	Found on the ventral midline 1 cun ventral to the border of the lower lip.

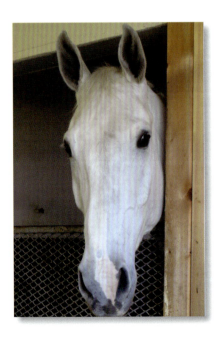

Governing Vessel
Du Mai
Yang Gathering Vessel

The Governing Vessel influences the yang channels and enhances the yang chi of the entire horse's body. Other specific attributes of the Governing Vessel are that it strengthens the spine, nourishes the brain, expels internal and external wind, and increases Kidney yang chi.

The acupoints of the Governing Vessel benefit the local areas and organs along its pathway. For example, Governing Vessel 4, *Gate of Vitality*, enhances Kidney function and strengthens the lower back. Many other energetics and functions are associated with each of the acupoints on the Governing Vessel.

In Chinese, this channel is called *Du Mai*. It absorbs, stores, and transfers yang chi in the same way the Conception Vessel serves as a reservoir and distribution system of yin chi for the 12 Major Meridians. The Governing Vessel provides the balance of yang chi throughout the meridian system.

Functions and Attributes

- Unites and balances yang chi within the 12 Major Meridians
- Governs the central nervous system
- Governs blood circulation
- Strengthens the spine
- Nourishes marrow and the brain
- Influences organs along the dorsal midline

Health Issues

- Autonomic nervous system issues
- Blood circulation problems
- External or internal invasion of wind
- Spinal pain or soreness
- Unconsciousness
- Respiratory emergency
- Kidney function problem

Emotional Issue

- Anxiety

Location and Flow of the Governing Vessel

The Governing Vessel meridian begins at the depression between the anus and the underside of the base of the tail, GV 1. A branch of the Governing Vessel extends to the tip of the tail. The major meridian travels along the dorsal midline toward the head and reaches GV 20 at the top of the head. It flows down the midline of the face and ends at GV 28, a point inside the upper gums.

NOTE: This meridian does not have a sister meridian; it runs along a single pathway on the body.

Governing Vessel Meridian

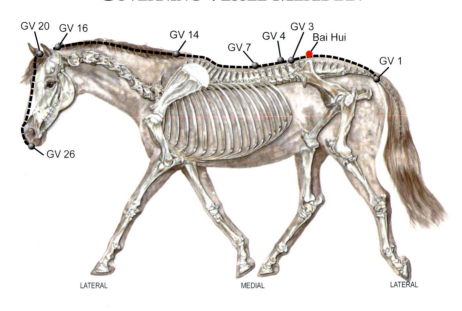

Point	Energetics/Function	Location
GV 1	Connecting point. Regulates the GV, calms the spirit, and strengthens the spinal column. **Benefits** spinal stiffness, lower back pain, seizures, diarrhea, or constipation.	Found on the dorsal midline in a depression between the anus and the base of the tail.
Bai Hui	Strengthens and warms Yang. **Benefits** any hindquarter pain or lameness, hip issues, colic, diarrhea, or overexertion.	Found on the dorsal midline at the lumbosacral space.
GV 3	Tonifies chi and Yang of Kidney, warms cold. **Benefits** lumbar disc issues, lower back pain, and pelvic limb paralysis.	Found on the dorsal midline in depression between lumbar vertebrae 4 and 5.
GV 4	Tonifies Kidney chi and Yang, Source chi, calms the spirit, restores Yang. **Benefits** bone disorders, Yang deficiency, intervertebral disc issues, seizures, infertility, and diarrhea.	Found on the dorsal midline in depression between lumbar vertebrae 2 and 3.
GV 7	Regulates the Spleen and Stomach. **Benefits** spinal stiffness and pain, and abdominal pain.	Found on the dorsal midline in the intervertebral space between thoracic vertebrae 17 and 18.

Governing Vessel Meridian

Point	Energetics/Function	Location
GV 14	Sea of Chi point. Clears Heat and dispels Wind. **Benefits** Yin deficiency, fever, cough, cervical pain, non-sweater, fever, heatstroke, and strengthens the immune system.	Found on the dorsal midline in depression between 7th cervical and 1st thoracic vertebrae, cranial to the highest point of the withers.
GV 16	Clears the brain, and opens the sensory orifices. **Benefits** intervertebral issues, mania, and seizure.	Found on the dorsal midline in a depression between the occipital protuberances, at the atlantooccipital joint.
GV 20	Clears the brain, calms the spirit, revives consciousness, restores collapsed Yang and counters prolapse. **Benefits** seizures, shock, neck stiffness, and shen disturbances.	Found on the dorsal midline at highest point of the poll.
GV 26	Clears the brain, calms the spirit, revives consciousness, restores collapsed Yang, regulates the GV and strengthens the back. **Benefits** emergencies such as shock, collapse, heatstroke, or coma. Helps the spine, and mania.	Found on the dorsal midline between the ventral limits of the nostrils.

Functions of the Meridian System

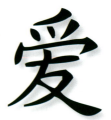

- The 12 Major Meridians are one continuous channel on which chi and blood (nourishing fluids) flow.

- Meridian energy shifts from yin to yang and yang to yin at the Jing-Well points located on the coronary bands.

- Meridians are relatively superficial, they flow between skin and muscle tissue.

- Each individual meridian is connected to a specific internal organ and communicates the energy of that organ to the surface of the horse's body.

- When performing an acupressure session, you are accessing the energy of the internal organs by "working" with the meridians on the surface of the horse's body.

The Meridian System is responsible for:

1. Communication between the *zang-fu* organs
2. Connection of the entire of the body
3. Circulation of chi, blood, and other vital substances

Chapter Nine

Assessing Your Horse

Horses can be tricksters. Hardwired not to exhibit any weakness, they'll do their best to stay up with the herd. When a horse is ill or injured in the wild, she's left behind to fend for herself because the leader can't allow the rest of his herd to become compromised. Her survival instincts dictate that she won't reveal she's in pain until she's desperately in pain. For you as a horse guardian, this predicament means you don't know your horse is experiencing pain during the early stages of a problem unless the situation involves an obvious traumatic event or sudden illness.

To add to the horse's predisposition to not show pain, repetitive injuries affecting the muscles, tendons, and ligaments are often difficult to detect because of their gradual onset. Suddenly, you're surprised to find your horse is lame. When this occurs, you've lost the opportunity to address the damage when it began and when it would have been much easier to resolve.

Then again, maybe your horse did give you subtle indicators he was not 100 percent sound. Watch for a change in attitude of any sort, which is often the first sign of a physical problem. The horse's inability to do something he did easily last week is not usually a case of needing more training or discipline; it probably means something hurts. Stumbling, shortness of breath, trouble turning, poor recovery from exercise, and, of course, any lameness are other tell-tale indicators that something's wrong.

Don't dismiss even a slight decline in your horse's performance. Even if it seems minor, pay attention to the hints your horse gives you. Tossing his head, refusing a jump, raspy sounding breathing, not being able to settle down while tacking up—any of these behaviors could mean something.

Many issues can affect equine performance. Every anatomical system has the potential to break down, whether it's from genetic problems, wear and tear, or stress. Issues of the musculoskeletal system aren't necessarily traumatic in nature. Degenerative joint disease (DJD), navicular syndrome, and various degrees of muscle soreness tend to have a gradual onset.

> **Traditional Chinese Medicine primarily involves preventive care.**

Traditional Chinese Medicine primarily involves preventive care. The intent is to avoid a pattern of disharmony and maintain a healthy, harmonious flow of chi and blood to enervate and nourish the horse's body. However, things happen—and not always what we want to have happen. Horses get injured. They get sick. And sometimes, it isn't clear exactly what's going on with your horse; you simply know he isn't quite right.

With an acute illness, injury, or any kind of health crisis, your holistic veterinarian is your first line of defense. Have your horse checked by a trusted healthcare professional before offering acupressure *unless* you're using acupoints that are specific emergency points before the veterinarian arrives.

Western medicine has excellent trauma care, sophisticated diagnostic tools, and surgical procedures that can save your horse's life. It's an important part of healthcare and, when used in conjunction with Chinese Medicine, can give your horse the best of both worlds.

TCM best serves you and your horse as a way to prevent disease and for chronic health issues. Once you've followed your vet's recommendations and acupressure is not contraindicated, you can proceed to use acupressure to restore your horse's balance so he can heal.

Assessment Process –The Four Examinations

Chinese medicine provides effective assessment tools to help identify your horse's health issue. The ancient Chinese medicine practitioners honed their five senses so they could assess human and animal conditions. The Four Examinations, also called The Four Pillars, rely on the practitioner's keen awareness of visual, auditory, olfactory, and touch indicators.

The Four Examinations include:
1. Observation
2. Listening and Smelling
3. Questions / Inquiry
4. Physical Palpation

Observation

According to Traditional Chinese Medicine, observation is "God-like." Why? Because it uses one's educated observation skills to see beyond the surface of the body once it's understood that internal activity is manifested externally (Law of Integrity).

Combined with the knowledge of yin-yang and *zang-fu* theories, observation is incredibly powerful and God-like in nature. We not only see how chi is functioning in the horse's body, we can interpret what we see using the guidance of yin-yang theory and knowledge of the functions and energetics of the *zang-fu* organs.

Here's an example of Observation. A young horse prances up to the fence line to greet you. His eye is bright and emanating curiosity; his coat is smooth and shiny. His muscles appear beautifully full and defined; his gait is even and lithe. Your impression is that he's vital, healthy, and happy.

Then, let's say, an older horse slowly walks up to the fence line. His eye is dull, there's no shine to his coat, he has minimal muscle tone, and his gait is uneven and plodding. You notice immediately this horse is not at the peak of his vitality and his health is questionable. You can see obvious visible indicators of declining health and a lack of vitality.

In the example just stated, the young horse can be said to have reasonably good balance of yin and yang. All his internal organs and processes must be functioning well because he's alert, moving well, and acting like a young horse. He gives no outward signs of any yin or yang imbalance; thus, his immune system is strong and external pathogens are not likely to invade his body. His *zang-fu* organs seem to be functioning, and his chi, blood, *shen* (spirit), and body fluids are harmoniously nourishing and invigorating his body.

On the other hand, the older horse demonstrates a lack of vitality. His eyes appear dull, his movements are ponderous and slow, his muscles are flaccid, and his coat is dull. This demonstrates a pattern of disharmony that tends to be cold in nature. Yin and yang aren't balanced. Because of his age and outward appearance, you can assume it has taken time for the horse to reach this state of ill health. His condition is chronic, and the external indicators point to a deficiency pattern of not enough heat and activity (yang) to balance the cold, damp, slower yin attributes.

Observation is crucial to the assessment process. The first observation is always overall appearance, conformation, vitality, responsiveness, and attitude. An initial general perception is followed by systematically examining the horse's eyes, nose, ears, mouth, tongue, gums, teeth, throat, limbs, nails, coat, and skin. The practitioner looks for discharges from the sensory orifices, lumps, rashes, masses, dryness, dampness, color of tissue—any indication of an imbalance of yin and yang in his body.

In TCM, practitioners heavily rely on tongue assessment. However, it's beyond the scope of this book to go into depth about the geography of the tongue or discuss different shapes, coatings, and colors in assessing and interpreting tongue indicators. Plus, it can be difficult to inspect a horse's tongue carefully. On an elementary level, though, a red tongue indicates a heat pattern, a pale tongue indicates an insufficiency of chi and blood, and a purple tongue indicates a stagnation of blood.

Listening and Smelling

The next phase relies on your senses of hearing and smelling. Listen to your horse's vocalizations, respiration, heart, and abdominal sounds. Is there any wheezing sound or congested breathing? Is his heart pounding loudly? Does his gut sound good? These are important indicators. Let's go into more detail.

Raspy or congested breathing could indicate a possible Lung imbalance. A rapid, pounding heart beat suggests a Heart or Pericardium imbalance. And, as every horse guardian knows, the lack of gut sounds isn't good. Stomach, Spleen, Small Intestine, and Large Intestine are the main organ systems responsible for taking in forage and water, breaking them down into absorbable nutrients, and ridding the body of waste. You should hear gut sounds of food moving through the horse's digestive tract.

Strong smells tend to be associated with excess heat syndromes. When the weather is warm, we can smell the sweet fragrance of a flower. On cold, chilly days, the flower may still be in bloom, but we're apt not to smell it. Body secretions and excretions have some smell but should not be extremely smelly.

Foul and sour body odors usually indicate retention of food. Specific odors are associated with each of the *zang* organs and can be used to ascertain the nature and origin of the imbalance the smell indicates. For instance, a heavy, overly-sweet fragrance is associated with a Stomach / Spleen, Earth Element imbalance.

Infections can smell and infections indicate excess heat. If your horse's manure has a burnt smell, this signifies a definite heat syndrome. Conversely, when manure has no smell, it could indicate a cold condition because manure ought to smell. No smell means the horse is not digesting well enough to break the forage down into nutrients. Essentially, his Stomach and Spleen aren't "cooking" his food because there's not enough heat, so this is considered a cold pattern.

Questions / Inquiry

It may seem strange to be asking yourself these questions if you're working with your own horse, but it's still a valuable process. Because you're familiar with your horse, you may have been overlooking important indicators. This process gives you an opportunity to ask good questions that clarify and expand your view.

With the current clinical signs gathered from Observation and Listening/Smelling in mind, start with general questions and progress to more specific ones to differentiate a particular pattern of disharmony:

- How old is your horse?
- Has your horse been neglected, abused, abandoned, or injured at any time?
- Does he have a friendly nature or is he aloof?
- Is he timid or fearful?
- How does he get along with other horses?
- Does he like humans besides you?
- Does he like cold weather or warm weather?
- In which season is he most active?
- What is his daily routine for feed, turn-out, exercise, and training?

- What is he fed?
- Is he on medications?
- Has he had medical procedures in the past?
- Has he received inoculations lately?
- How often is he wormed?
- Does he get supplements? If so, which ones and why?
- Have there been any changes in his environment recently?

You could continue to ask many more questions, but this is a good start in knowing your horse's general daily existence. Now list any clinical signs of his current condition:

- Is your horse in pain or showing signs of weakness?
- Has he had any recent changes in behavior?
- Is he showing signs of stress or obsessive behaviors?
- Is he restless or lethargic? If so, at what time of day is he more restless or uncomfortable?

A picture should be forming about your horse's lifestyle and how he's coping within his environment. You need to understand his nature as well as his exposure to external factors and internal stressors related to his current condition.

All of these inquiries are part of the puzzle for understanding your horse's condition. With Eastern medicine, you want to have as full a picture as possible because the acupoints selected for the session need to be specific for your horse.

If you suspect your horse has been exposed to toxic chemicals, his condition is deteriorating, or if he displays a sudden change in behavior, have a veterinarian check him immediately. Remember, acupressure is a complementary therapy, not a substitute for veterinary care.

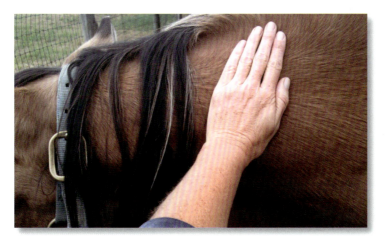

Physical Palpation

Start by literally touching your horse all over his body from head to hind hooves. It's good to feel your horse all over to get a sense of his body, if he's comfortable with touch. Feel for:

- Temperature to consider chi flow,
- Muscle tension to understand potential loss of blood and chi flow,
- Lumps that may be swelling or edema or a mass,
- Moisture levels, and
- Tender areas.

All of these are important for the fourth phase of the Four Examinations. All palpation should be reasonably gentle because you don't want to "spank the crying baby" and cause further pain or injury.

It's wise to write down what you are feeling so you can keep track of it. The moment you place your hands on your horse, you're changing the energy of the horse's body. Your hands bring more chi and blood to wherever you place them, no matter what. This is how acupressure works. Your touch is going to influence the horse's body, and you've actually begun the acupressure session just by touching him.

Like observing the tongue in Chinese medicine, pulses are used extensively in the assessment process. Pulses are usually taken bilaterally along the carotid artery on the ventral side of the horse's neck.

Although pulses are an important part of physical palpation, teaching them in an introductory book wouldn't be appropriate because it takes years of conscientious practice to become proficient at taking pulses. The practitioner is feeling for a particular location of a pulse that corresponds to specific organ systems. Then the practitioner determines whether the pulses are superficial or deep, rapid or slow, strong or weak, wide or narrow, thick or wiry, and many other qualities a pulse can express.

The highly detailed, wonderful study of pulses requires years of training because in TCM, both taking and interpreting pulses become complex. To greatly simplify for introductory purposes, however, a rapid pulse usually indicates a heat syndrome, while a slow pulse indicates a cold syndrome.

Association and Alarm Points

Two acupoint classifications are commonly used to help assess a horse during the Physical Palpation phase of the Four Examinations because they provide information about how the *zang-fu* organs are functioning. By palpating the Association points along the horse's back on the Bladder meridian, you can learn how the internal organs "feel." When one of the Association points feels warm or cool to the touch, you can check the corresponding Alarm point to see how deeply an imbalance has penetrated the body. Here's how it works in more detail.

The Association Points, or Back Transporting, or Back-*Shu* Points are located along the medial (close to the spine) channel of the Bladder Meridian. Each of the Association Points is directly related to the *zang-fu* organ for which it's named. Because of this internal-external relationship with each of the organ systems, these points can communicate the condition of each for assessment purposes.

For instance, hold the soft tip of your thumb at a 45- to 90-degree angle to the horse's body on Bladder 13 (Bl 13), which is the Lung Association point. Feel if the point is hot, cold, sinking, protruding, reactive, or normal. If Bl 13 feels cold and lifeless, there could be an imbalance in the Lung organ system (i.e., the Lung organ itself and the meridian) of a cold nature.

ASSOCIATION POINTS

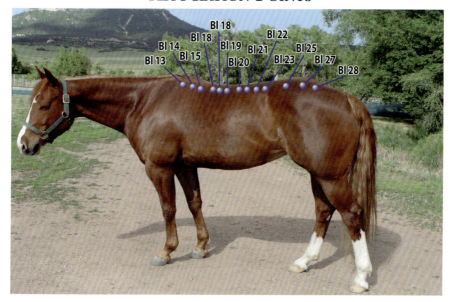

Point Location

BL 13	Three cun lateral to the dorsal midline in the 8th intercostal space.
Bl 14	Three cun lateral to the dorsal midline in the 9th intercostal space.
Bl 15	Three cun lateral to the dorsal midline in the 10th intercostal space.
Bl 18	3 cun lateral to the dorsal midline in the 13th and 14th intercostal spaces.
Bl 19	Three cun lateral to the dorsal midline in the 15th intercostal space.
Bl 20	Three cun lateral to the dorsal midline in the last (17th) intercostal space.
Bl 21	Three cun lateral to the dorsal midline caudal to the last rib.
Bl 22	Three cun lateral to dorsal midline between 1st and 2nd lumbar vertebrae.
Bl 23	Three cun lateral to the dorsal midline between the 2nd and 3rd lumbar vertebrae, directly dorsal to the ventral end of the last rib.
Bl 25	Three cun lateral to dorsal midline between 1st and 2nd sacral vertebrae.
Bl 27	Three cun lateral to dorsal midline between 1st and 2nd sacral vertebrae.
Bl 28	Three cun lateral to the dorsal midline between the 2nd and 3rd sacral vertebrae.

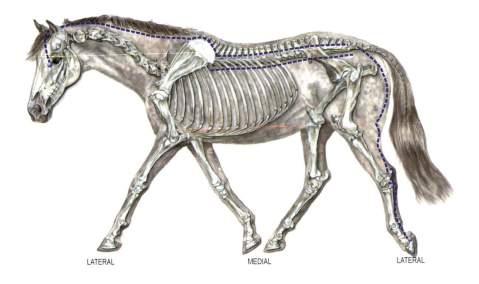

LATERAL   MEDIAL   LATERAL

Another example: Bladder 14 (Bl 14) is the Back-*Shu* point for the Pericardium, the sac surrounding the heart. When other indicators point to an imbalance in the Pericardium, you can check Bl 14 to detect if your horse is reactive or if you can feel any heat, coolness, softness, hardness, sinking, or anything other than a smooth and even feeling. Information during the palpation phase of the Four Examinations provides one more indicator of an imbalance related to a particular organ system and its nature.

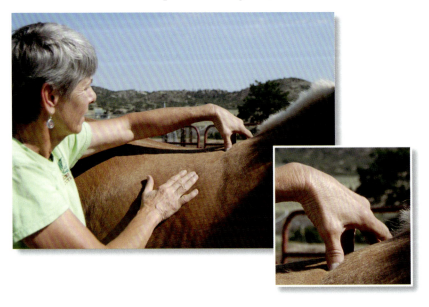

Proceed checking each of the Association points along the Bladder meridian. Make note of any of the acupoints that feel something other than normal.

Alarm Points, or Front-*Mu* Points, further identify the depth and nature of an imbalance within a specific organ system. The Alarm points are found on the ventral (underside) or ventrolateral (lower side) aspect of the horse's trunk. These acupoints are where chi of a *zang-fu* organ accumulates when the organ itself is suffering from an imbalance. Once the imbalance or disease has reached the *zang-fu* organs, the horse will most likely react to thumb pressure on these points.

When the Association point for the Lung (Bl 13) is reactive or indicates an imbalance in any way, the practitioner checks Lung 1 (Lu 1) to ascertain if the imbalance has gone beyond the meridian level of the animal and is affecting the Lung organ. The Alarm points tell you if there's organ involvement in the imbalance you detected from the Association point.

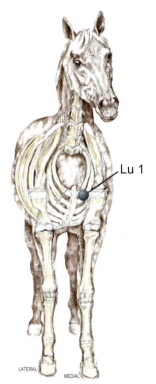

You notice your horse has yellow nasal discharge and his breathing sounds congested, so you check Bl 13, the Lung Association point, to assess the imbalance in the entire organ system. Bl 13 feels cool to the touch. You then check Lu 1, the Lung Alarm point, to see if there's Lung organ involvement in the imbalance or if the problem is manifesting only superficially as a Lung meridian imbalance. If it's only the Association point that feels cool and your horse has no response when you touch Lu 1, the Alarm point, you know the Lung imbalance hasn't penetrated deeply and affected the Lung organ.

Alarm Points

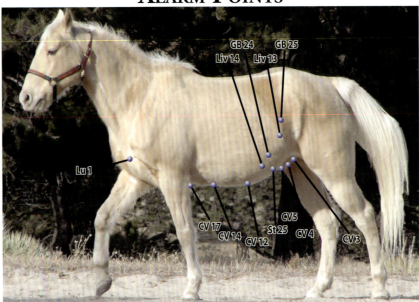

Point   Location

Lu 1 — Alarm point for the Lung. In depression in the center of the muscle belly of the descending pectoral muscle at the level of the 1st intercostal space.

St 25 — Alarm point for the Large Intestine. Located 2 cun lateral to the umbilicus.

CV 12 — Alarm point for the Stomach. On ventral midline, halfway between the xiphoid process and the umbilicus.

Liv 13 — Alarm point for the Spleen. Found on the lateral side of abdomen on the lower margin of the 2nd to the last rib.

CV 14 — Alarm point for the Heart. Ventral midline at level of the xiphoid process.

CV 4 — Alarm point for the Small Intestine. Found on the ventral midline 3 cun caudal to the umbilicus.

CV 3 — Alarm point for the Bladder. Ventral midline 4 cun caudal to the umbilicus.

GB 25 — Alarm point of Kidney. Located at the caudal border of the last rib.

CV 17 — Alarm point for the Pericardium. Found on the ventral midline at the level of the caudal border of the elbow.

CV 5 — Alarm point for the Triple Heater. Ventral midline 2 cun caudal to umbilicus.

GB 24 — Alarm point for GB. At the 14th intercostal space, caudal & dorsal to Liv 14.

Liv 14 — Alarm point for Liver. At 13th intercostal space at the level of the elbow.

Both the Association and Alarm points provide invaluable information for assessing a horse's condition because they narrow the imbalance to particular organ systems and provide indicators regarding the nature of the imbalance.

The Four Examinations may seem a bit crude because they rely on the human senses, but practitioners who become proficient in each of these assessment techniques can often detect sub-clinical health issues. The whole process can yield an extremely thorough and accurate assessment.

Quick Review of the Assessment Process

Taking it from the top:

Observe your horse with a critical eye. Any discharges? Is his eye bright? How's his weight? What's his general conformation and attitude? Is his muscle tone good? What does his manure look like? Watch him walk and trot. What do you see? Are there any indications of a recent injury?

Listen to detect anything unusual about his vocalizations. Does his breathing sound clear? Can you hear his gut sounds? How do his hoof-steps sound when he walks on a hard surface?

Smell to see if your horse has a sweet grassy smell. Does he smell about the same from front to back? How does his breath smell? Any indication of infection? How does his manure smell?

Question/Inquiry as you go through an inventory of your horse's life. What's his daily routine? Examine his exercise, training, feed, turn-out, socializing, likes and dislikes, best time of the year, supplements, medications, procedures, vaccines, worming schedule, environment, and anything else that influences his health and well-being today.

Palpate whatever parts of your horse you're led to feel. By the time you get to this fourth phase of the Four Examinations, you should have a hunch or two about what you want to check out when you touch your horse.

Go over his whole body feeling for hot or cold areas, lumps and bumps, and places to which he reacts. Record your findings and move on to the

Association points. If Bladder 18 (Bl 18), the Liver Association point, feels warm, go to Liver 14 (Liv 14), the Liver **Alarm point**, to assess if the Liver organ is involved in the imbalance. If your horse reacts to your touching Liv 14, then you know you need to help resolve a Liver organ imbalance.

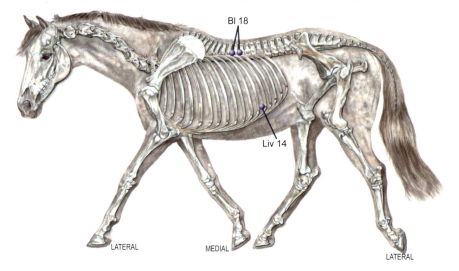

It may seem like a lot to do! But think of all you'll learn about your horse. Now that you've gathered all this information, how are you going to interpret it and work with it? What does it mean?

Interpretation for Assessment Purposes

When you're learning something new, it's best to begin by taking small steps. Chinese medicine can be extremely complex. Like anything else, the more you learn and know, the more you can refine your approach to the subject matter. The beauty of Chinese medicine is you can take a simple approach and still benefit your horse.

In gathering all this detailed information about your horse, you're figuring out if he's experiencing any *zang-fu* organ system imbalances, presenting with any disease, or suffering from a musculoskeletal issue. You've checked your horse from top to bottom, and now you have to see how to resolve a physical or emotional issue.

Consider the functions and energetics of the *zang-fu* organs and their meridians. Say your horse has an inflamed tendon. Tendons are associated with the Liver. You can use acupoints for the Liver and Gall Bladder, the Liver's paired yang organ, to help reduce the inflammation. Acupoints commonly used for tendon issues are Liver 2 and 3 (Liv 2 and 3), and Gall Bladder 34 (GB 34), the Influential point for tendons and ligaments.

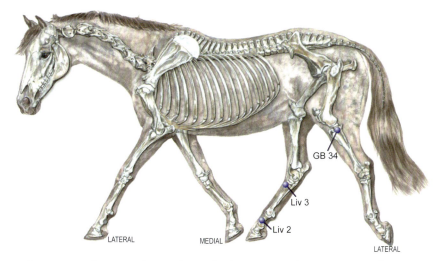

Another example: Your horse has whole grain in his manure. The grain is not being broken down into bio-absorbable nutrients because the Stomach and Spleen don't have enough heat to cook the grain properly. This indicates a Stomach-Spleen imbalance. To resolve this digestion problem, you will have to select acupoints known to restore balance to Stomach and Spleen chi. Acupoints often used to work with this imbalance are Stomach 36 (St 36), Spleen 6 (Sp 6), and Conception Vessel 12 (CV 12).

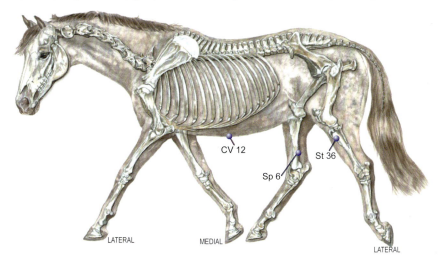

If your horse has dry, flaky skin, there's not enough moisture getting to the surface of his skin. Dry, flaky skin is seen in Chinese medicine as a blood deficiency because blood carries moisture and nutrients needed for healthy skin. The Lung governs skin and is associated with body fluids, and the Heart circulates blood. Your objective in creating an acupressure session is to select acupoints that will support and balance Lung and Heart function.

Compare the clinical signs your horse is exhibiting to the job the organ system does in the body to figure out what kind of imbalance your horse is presenting. Of course we hope that most of the time your horse is in great shape. Then the best acupressure session you can offer him is an Immune System Strengthening session to be found in the Specific Conditions chapter of this book. Better to support his health and well-being consistently than to have to deal with resolving imbalances.

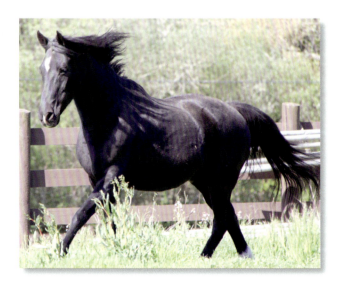

Chapter Ten

EQUINE ACUPRESSURE SESSION PROTOCOL

Horses are sensitive, intelligent animals. Today, their adaptability and capacity to learn has made them an ideal companion in human therapeutic assistance and sport. It's gratifying to be able to offer our horses an acupressure session that's truly beneficial for them. Equine acupressure is gentle, yet powerful and horses are incredibly responsive. This chapter carries you further into the journey of helping your horse feel his best.

When you begin the acupressure session, the most important element is for you to be mentally present. Your horse is highly aware of your mental state. In fact, it can be scary to think how attuned your horse is to your energy. Take your mind off him for an instant and he knows it; his behavior can change in a flash.

An acupressure session is a dynamic, energetic interaction between two equal partners—you and your horse. Your role as a partner in the acupressure session is to bring the clear intention of enhancing the horse's health and well-being. When planning your acupressure session, you need to clear your mind, breathe, and use your knowledge, experience, and intuition. The other half of the partnership is your horse. He brings his innate ability to feel energetic sensations and assist in the balancing process.

> **An acupressure session is a dynamic, energetic interaction between two equal partners — you and your horse.**

Don't be disturbed if your horse doesn't display his pleasure or internal sensory experience during an acupressure session. Lots of horses will walk away and shake after the session to help integrate the energy work you've just done. Then again, other horses are quite expressive throughout the entire session, especially as they become more familiar with enjoying an acupressure session.

Watching your horse when he's feeling good is a rich experience. However, working with his body can be humbling. Remember—if the body can heal, it will. This means if the horse is sick or injured, he will benefit from an acupressure session to the level his body is capable of healing at that time. Because only the body can heal itself, your job is to create the "environment" in which his body has the best opportunity to heal.

No form of medicine can claim to cure an illness. You can only apply techniques and remedies and hope that the body is able to respond positively. At times, a disease has penetrated deeply into the body and either yin or yang chi has been irreparably damaged. In this circumstance, you want to provide your horse with consistent acupressure sessions to manage his condition and have him be as comfortable and active as possible.

Acupressure has a significant place in the spectrum of animal care. Domesticated horses have to adapt to situations that are far removed from their natural regimen and environment. The amazing thing is, horses do adapt and survive—but at what cost? Acupressure can help relieve some of the stress they have to contend with by living among us. Each session provides you and your horse an important time to connect, while allowing stress to fall away so the two of you can develop a caring space where healing can occur.

Acupressure Protocol

During your grooming routine after riding is often a good time to include an acupressure session. It's a way to communicate your caring intentions through intentional touch. Your horse knows the difference between grooming and touch with the intention of helping him balance his internal chi and nourish his body. Horses are keenly aware of their energetics.

It's interesting to see how once your horse trusts your intentions, she may come to expect an acupressure session. A lot of horses even tell you with their nose which acupoints they want you to stimulate. It's exciting when you become real partners in the process.

The acupressure session protocol includes three major segments: Pre-Session, Session, and Post-Session. Within each major segment are specific tasks leading you to the next portion of the session. This protocol creates a context for healing and balancing to maintain or restore the harmonious flow of chi and blood.

Pre-Session

Selecting a Location. Ideally, find a familiar place where you and your horse are safe and comfortable. It's good for the horse to be able to move around a bit during the session. Make sure your safety isn't in jeopardy. It's best to have someone holding his lead, but if that's not possible, a single loose tie will work.

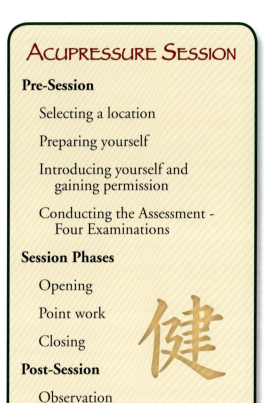

You may be in the midst of a show, in a busy barn, or in another environment where there are other horses and people. You want to find a space where you'll have the fewest distractions possible, but it would be unrealistic to expect none at all. When there's activity, remember to face your horse toward whatever is happening so he can see what's going on and isn't surprised by the commotion.

Preparing Yourself. Your healing intent has a tremendous impact on an acupressure session. As you prepare to offer your horse a session, take a few minutes to get in touch with your own energy and formulate your intention for the session.

Try this breathing exercise: Let all of life's pressures and concerns fall away. Take six to eight deep, even breaths and allow yourself to exhale down to the bottom of your breath. As you exhale, follow the vibration of your breath as it moves away from you. Feel yourself release any tension in your body. If thoughts of your grocery list arise, just breathe them away. Then take your next three breaths and focus on your heart opening to your highest intent. Your job is to *be there* for your horse at this moment.

Formulating your *healing intention* for the session is essential to a successful outcome. Take a few minutes to focus on your horse and think about how you want him to feel his best physically and emotionally. The quality of the session is greatly enhanced by your healing intent. Do you want your horse to heal from a specific illness or injury? Are you most interested in his remaining balanced and healthy? Your intention provides the impetus for the entire acupressure session.

Introducing Yourself and Gaining Permission. It might seem strange to introduce yourself to your own horse, but what you're doing is asking your horse if he would like to join you in an acupressure session. Most horses have good manners. They're highly respectful of personal space, especially when they've had a good mother who taught them the ways of horses. Humans need to be equally respectful.

Rather than assuming your horse wants you to work on him, let him know you're available to work *with* him. You can do this verbally, nonverbally, or even project a mental picture. Horses understand these forms of communication when you mean them sincerely.

Look for signals that tell you your horse is giving you permission to touch him. These signals can take a variety of forms, such as turning toward you, leaning into you, softening his eye, showing you an acupoint he wants you to work on, or communicating energetically. If your horse doesn't give you a response, try moving to another location and ask for permission again. If, after three attempts to work with him, he's still unresponsive, honor his choice not to have an acupressure session at that time. Ask again some other day.

Conducting the Assessment – Four Examinations.

The assessment process blends seamlessly into the acupressure session. The assessment process during the pre-session is more like a first impression. Then as you progress into assessing your horse, you shift to a higher level of detail when checking for clinical signs of imbalance. This more critical step takes you into the Opening phase of the acupressure session.

The second you look at your horse, you're probably getting an idea of how he's doing. When his eye is bright, his conformation looks good, and his attitude emanates vitality, you know he's ready to have fun. When he's slow moving and showing no interest in anything, it's clear he's not feeling well.

This first impression can tell you a lot, but you need to go further and gather more detailed information. This is when you begin the Four Examinations discussed in the assessment chapter (Chapter Nine). Observation, Listening/Smelling, and Questions are usually seen as part of the Pre-Session assessment process. Take your time to go through each one of these "examinations" in detail. Write down your findings so you have a record of what you detected. Indicators of a potential pattern of disharmony are an important part of a picture you're forming about your horse.

Session Phases

Opening. Because few hard lines of division exist between one phase of the acupressure protocol and the next, the acupressure session begins with the fourth phase of the Four Examinations, the Physical Palpation segment. The reason the physical is included in the Opening Phase of the acupressure session is that when you touch your horse, you've begun balancing chi and blood. Simply by virtue of your touch, the horse's energetic balance starts to shift. The Opening Phase marks the moment you narrow your focus and begin to identify, or discern, specific issues related to the indicators your horse is exhibiting.

> **Simply by virtue of your touch, the horse's energetic balance starts to shift.**

Let's review for a minute. When performing the Four Examinations during the Pre-Session, you're collecting information that can be gathered from external manifestations. You're using your observation skills: How is his conformation? Is his movement fluid? Is he weighting one leg more than the other? Are his hooves healthy? Any coat issues? Can you detect any unusual discharges? Jot down everything you notice.

Next, you listen to respiration, vocalization, and gut sounds. This is followed by smelling to detect any heat syndrome such as an infection that could be happening. Add any more indicators you find to your log.

Run through a series of questions about your horse's daily routine. Think about any medications, inoculations, or medical procedures he has had. History? Supplements? Injuries? Write everything down so you have a record and good picture of your horse.

Now the Opening begins. You are ready for the general hands-on portion of the assessment process. Feel for temperature changes all over your horse's body. How do his muscles feel? Are there any lumps? Swelling? Edema? Write down anything you feel.

During this process you're forming an idea of what's going on with your horse. If he's moving well, his attitude is good, muscle tone is good, flexibility is wonderful, temperature all over is fine—that's great. It's time to perform a sweep along the Bladder meridian.

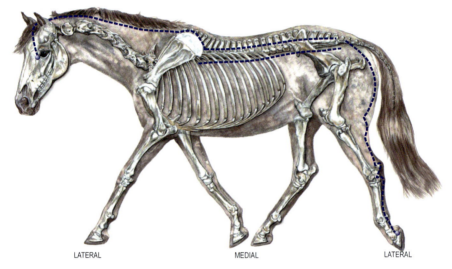

LATERAL   MEDIAL   LATERAL

You are tracing the Bladder meridian to let your horse know you're doing something other than grooming or patting him. You're preparing him for *intentional touch*. The acupressure session has begun and you're shifting your attention and intention.

The Bladder meridian is located on the dorsal aspect, or back, of the horse approximately one hand-width off the spine. Though the Bladder meridian begins at the inner corner, or inner canthus, of the eye bilaterally, you can start tracing the meridian on the horse's neck where it's easier to reach. Glide the heel of your hand slowly and evenly along the Bladder meridian, feeling for hot or cold areas and hard or soft spots. Rest your other hand comfortably somewhere on the horse's body. The resting hand serves as an anchor that connects you with the horse and can help you feel the horse's reaction to the hand tracing the meridian.

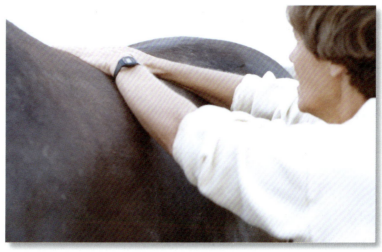
Work along the Bladder meridian feeling for hot and cold spots.

Continue tracing the Bladder meridian down the horse's back toward the tail, staying about one hand-width off his spine. Continue down the hind leg on the caudolateral aspect and finish on the back of the coronary band. Repeat this procedure, starting on the neck and tracing the meridian three times on each side of your horse.

While performing the Opening by tracing the Bladder meridian, pay attention to the temperature of each section of your horse's back. The temperature can offer a glimpse of what could be occurring internally. For instance, it can communicate how well the Heart is circulating chi and blood.

If your horse has just been exercising, his muscles are probably going to be warm from exertion. This is not an imbalance. However, it's important to note if your horse has been standing around and not exercising and he feels hot along his neck, withers, back, or hind legs. The presence of heat in that situation likely indicates an imbalance.

Older horses may feel cool in the loin area, for instance, indicating a possible imbalance related to the Kidney meridian. This does not mean something dire, such as kidney disease; it could simply be an imbalance that can be easily resolved or managed by selecting acupoints that enhance Kidney chi to warm the loin.

> **Words in Eastern medicine convey very different meanings than in conventional Western medicine.**

Words in Eastern medicine convey very different meanings than in conventional Western medicine. In Eastern medicine, the concepts are different and when we refer to the word *Kidney*, we're conceiving of a host of energetics and body functions, not just the physical kidneys. The implications are quite different. When identifying an imbalance or a pattern of disharmony, we have to be careful not to sound alarms by using words for which others may not have the same frame of reference.

Saying there's heat along the Bladder meridian near the kidneys might scare someone; better to follow through with the complete Opening before jumping to conclusions. It could be as simple as a chi and blood imbalance that disappears after the Opening because you've begun the balancing process.

On the other hand, at times you may discover an inflammation, an injury, or a disease pattern of disharmony that needs veterinary attention. It's important to know when to call your holistic veterinarian. It's a judgment call; however, seek veterinary care if there's even the slightest thought that the horse should be seen by a vet, please be sure to call. Have your vet come out or follow the vet's recommendation before proceeding with an acupressure session. Always have the best interest of the horse firmly in mind.

As you trace the Bladder meridian three times on each side of your horse, note any temperature changes, sensitivities, lumps, indents, protrusions, soft or hard areas. At this moment during the Opening procedure, write down what you feel and where it's located, because the next step in the process can yield more definitive information.

Association Points, Back Shu Points

Continue the assessment process using the Association points (or Back *Shu* points) along the Bladder meridian. The Association points (discussed in the assessment chapter) include a classification of acupoints that share the attribute of being internally connected with the *zang-fu* organ for which they are named. These points are used during the Opening because they can indicate how the organ system is functioning. If the Association point feels cold, then there may be other indicators pointing to an imbalance within that meridian or the organ itself.

Association Points

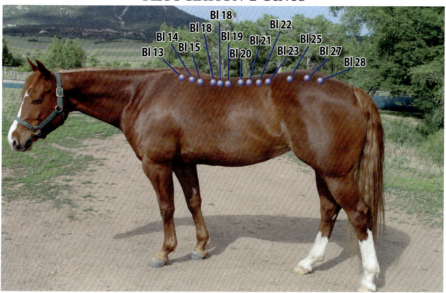

Point	Location
BL 13	Three cun lateral to the dorsal midline in the 8th intercostal space.
Bl 14	Three cun lateral to the dorsal midline in the 9th intercostal space.
Bl 15	Three cun lateral to the dorsal midline in the 10th intercostal space.
Bl 18	3 cun lateral to the dorsal midline in the 13th and 14th intercostal spaces.
Bl 19	Three cun lateral to the dorsal midline in the 15th intercostal space.
Bl 20	Three cun lateral to the dorsal midline in the last (17th) intercostal space.
Bl 21	Three cun lateral to the dorsal midline caudal to the last rib.
Bl 22	Three cun lateral to dorsal midline between 1st and 2nd lumbar vertebrae.
Bl 23	Three cun lateral to the dorsal midline between the 2nd and 3rd lumbar vertebrae, directly dorsal to the ventral end of the last rib.
Bl 25	Three cun lateral to dorsal midline between 1st and 2nd sacral vertebrae.
Bl 27	Three cun lateral to dorsal midline between 1st and 2nd sacral vertebrae.
Bl 28	Three cun lateral to dorsal midline between 2nd and 3rd sacral vertebrae.

Additionally, the Association point on one side of your horse may not feel the same on the opposite side. Think of these points as providing one more piece of information to add to other indicators gathered during the Four Examinations.

Technique

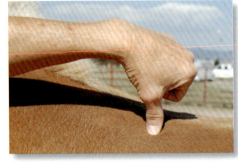

To begin, use the soft tip of your thumb at a 45° to 90° angle to the surface of the horse's back and apply gentle pressure. There's no need to press down hard because the acupoint is just beneath the surface of the skin. In fact, you often feel more when you don't press deeply. Feel each one of the 12 Association points, starting with Bladder 13, the Association point for the Lung. Note temperature and texture differences of the points. It is important to be conscious of any sensitivity to a specific point your horse may have. Then move on to the next acupoint.

The Association point for the Pericardium (i.e., the sac surrounding and protecting the Heart located in the thoracic region of the horse's body) is Bladder 14 (Bl 14). Say your horse reacts when you touch the point with the soft tip of your thumb and Bl 14 feels warmer than the surrounding area. Additionally, you've noticed your horse seems apprehensive and wary of strangers. Plus, his body language and the look in his eye tell you he's being overly self-protective. These are all indicators your horse is having trust issues. Trust is related to the functioning of the Pericardium. Combine this information with Bl 14 feeling warm. Given his behavior and the feeling of the point, you know the Pericardium is experiencing some level of imbalance.

Continue to feel each one of the 12 Association points on one side, then repeat checking the Association points on the opposite side of your horse. Remember, each of these acupoints is an external connection with each of the 12 internal organ systems. This means you are actually feeling what may be occurring within the organ system. It's important to be conscious of any sensitivity to a specific point your horse may have. Record anything you detect.

When you're learning, this process seems to take a long time and requires a lot of concentration. True, it does at first. With practice, you'll become familiar with the assessment process and it will go more quickly and smoothly.

Alarm Points, Front *Mu* Points

Going back to the example of the Pericardium imbalance: You know there's an imbalance because your horse is behaving warily and Bladder 14 (Bl 14) feels warmer than the rest of his body. Now you need to check the Alarm point for the Pericardium. By checking the Alarm point, you will find out how deeply into the body the imbalance has gone. If your horse shows no sign of discomfort or the Alarm point feels consistent with the rest of his body, it means the imbalance hasn't affected the Pericardium itself. The imbalance is more superficial and is only an imbalance along the Pericardium meridian. Because it's relatively superficial, it will be easier to resolve.

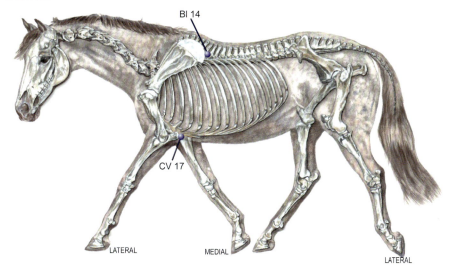

Bladder 14 (Bl 14), Association point for the Pericardium
Conception Vessel 17 (CV 17), Alarm point for the Pericardium

The Alarm point for the Pericardium is Conception Vessel 17 (CV 17). When you palpate this point very gently, let's say your horse reacts by moving away from you. This reaction indicates that the Pericardium is more deeply impacted by the imbalance and it's affecting the internal organ itself. When this happens, it will take longer to resolve your horse's trust issue. It will require a longer-term, consistent approach that could include other modalities along with acupressure.

Here's an example: Your 18-year old mare has been slowing down considerably the past three months. Your vet has done an exam and she checked out fine. You've been giving her an Immune System Strengthening acupressure session every week, and she seems to perk up for a few days after each session. You've noticed that she's fussy under saddle and a bit cold in the loin area. When you checked Bladder 23 (Bl 23), Association point for Kidney, it was definitely cool to the touch. When you lightly touched the Alarm point for Kidney, Gall Bladder 25 (GB 25), she stepped away from you. All of these indicators—slowing down, uncomfortable under saddle, cool along the loin, Bl 23 feeling cool, and GB 25 being reactive—point to a Kidney imbalance affecting the entire Kidney organ system.

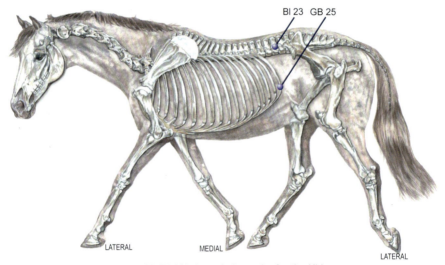

Bladder 23 (Bl 23), Association point for the Kidney
Gall Bladder 25 (GB 25), Alarm point for the Kidney

One more example: A young mare has a drippy nose, her breathing sounds congested, and she has absolutely no interest in going on a trail ride. She's usually the life of the ride, but today she wants to stay in her paddock. Upon checking her Association points, Bladder 13 (Bl 13), the Association point for the Lung, feels slightly sunken and cool. The Lung Alarm point, Lung 1 (Lu 1) feels fine and the mare shows no reaction. She's exhibiting a common cold, called Excess Wind-Cold in Chinese medicine.

This Excess Wind-Cold condition will last a short time and, most likely, won't affect the Lung organ. It's considered superficial in nature and can be managed on the meridian level. An acupressure session to address this condition will focus on supporting the Lung to balance the Lung meridian.

Acupoint Selection

Now that you've gathered a lot of information about your horse and her condition, if there are no specific emotional or physical issues, it's always good to offer your horse an Immune System Strengthening acupressure session (see chart in Chapter Eleven). Every horse on earth can benefit from having her immune system supported.

If you've identified a few issues you'd like to address with an acupressure session, decide which issue is most pressing or causing your horse the most discomfort. Once you've selected the emotional or physical issue you want to address first, review the functions of the *zang-fu* organ system to figure out which organ system is exhibiting a pattern of disharmony.

For instance, you notice your mare's eyes are tearing excessively and there's no evidence of an inflammation or infection—no heat or yellow discharge are present. You check the Association points, and Bladder 18 (Bl 18), the Liver Association point, feels a bit cool. Then you check the Liver Alarm point, Liver 14 (Liv 14), and it feels fine and your mare doesn't react. When you look at the functions of the *zang-fu* organ systems, you learn that eyes are the sensory organ associated with Liver. You conclude she has a mild Liver imbalance of a cold nature.

What acupoints can you use to help resolve this Liver imbalance? Some point selection techniques are complicated, while others are quite simple. To introduce you to acupoint selection, let's start with a simple and direct method of selecting acupoints.

The Association points used during the assessment portion of the Opening are powerful acupoints because they're internally and externally connected to an organ. Association points can be of great benefit during the acupressure session as well as the assessment. For the Liver imbalance, you can select Bladder 18 (Bl 18), the Liver Association point for two (bilateral) of the points for your acupressure session.

Combining Association points with another category of points called Source, or *Yuan*, points creates a simple, yet powerful selection of acupoints for the Point Work segment of the acupressure session.

Each of the 12 Major Meridians has its own Source point. Source chi is original essence chi that the horse inherits from the dam and sire; it's the Original chi with which the animal arrives on earth. Basically, if the dam is an Arabian and the sire is an Arabian, the offspring is going to be an Arabian. This is the foal's source, or original, chi. When using Source points, you are accessing and stimulating the essence and fundamental chi for your horse.

Another significant energetic characteristic of Source points is that when they're palpated, they do what's necessary to balance the organ system. Source points respond to what the body needs at the time and you don't have to be concerned whether the condition is excess or deficient in nature. This is a significant attribute, especially when you're just learning acupressure.

To select the appropriate Source point to resolve the Liver imbalance, you look at the Source point chart and find the Liver Source point, Liver 3 (Liv 3). This point is located on the hind leg, and you will apply finger pressure to stimulate Liver 3 on both the right and left hind legs.

The acupoints you've selected to balance the mare's Liver and resolve excess tearing are Bladder 18, the Liver Association point and Liver 3, the Source point on the Liver meridian. You're going to palpate these points on both sides of your horse. The Point Work segment of your acupressure session will therefore have four acupoints.

Point selection for a horse with problems digesting forage could be the Spleen Association point, Spleen 20 (Sp 20) and the Source point for Spleen, Spleen 3 (Sp 3). The Spleen is responsible for creating the "rotting and ripening" (fermentation process) in the horse's Stomach and digestive tract. The acupressure session includes four acupoints because these points are bilateral.

For an inhalant allergy to dust, you can select Bladder 13 (Bl 13), the Association point for Lung, and Lung 9 (Lu 9), the Source point for Lung. Palpate these points on both sides of your horse to support your horse's Lung function.

SOURCE POINTS

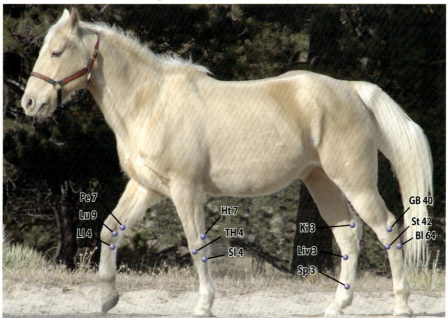

Point   Location

Lu 9   Middle of medial aspect of foreleg, on radial side of the carpus, between 1st and 2nd row of carpal bones just cranial to accessory carpal bone.

LI 4   Found distal and medial to the head of the medial splint bone.

St 42   Distal to the hock joint on the craniolateral aspect of the metatarsus.

Sp 3   Found on the distal end of the medial splint bone.

Ht 7   On caudolateral aspect of radius proximal to accessory carpal bone.

SI 4   On the lateral surface of the forelimb, at level of the lateral splint bone.

Bl 64   Located caudodistal to the head of the lateral splint bone.

Ki 3   Found in the depression between the medial malleolus of the tibia and the tendocalcaneus. Opposite Bl 60.

Pe 7   At the level of the accessory carpal bone on medial aspect of the foreleg.

TH 4   In depression slightly lateral to middle of the cranial surface of carpal joint, between intermediate and 3rd carpal bones.

GB 40   Craniodistal to tip of lateral malleolus of tibia over the tendon of lateral digital extensor.

Liv 3   Craniodistal aspect of cannon bone at level of head of medial splint bone.

Association and Source points make for a good acupressure session that's focused directly on the clinical sign the horse is presenting. In Chapter Eleven, you'll find charts and suggested acupoints for specific common equine conditions. After thousands of years of clinical observation, Traditional Chinese Medicine practitioners have determined the functions and energetics of acupoints. The acupoints presented are known to have a particular effect to help resolve the condition.

When learning how to select acupoints, it can be very helpful to refer to specific condition charts. It's another approach to helping your horse feel his best.

Point Selection Process

Assessment
- **Four Examinations**
  - Observation
  - Listening / Smelling
  - Inquiry / Questions
  - Physical palpation
    - General physical
    - Association points
    - Alarm points

Assessment Outcome
- Current condition
- Identify meridian(s) / Organ system involvement

Point Selection
- Association point(s)
- Source point(s)

Point Work. It takes practice to educate your hands. By educating your hands, we mean tuning in and being able to focus on the sensations your hands and fingers are experiencing during the initial general physical, Association points, Point Work, and the last segment of the acupressure session, the Closing. Becoming conscious of temperature changes and shifts in texture requires considerable effort. In time and with practice, you will be able to actually feel chi moving under your fingers telling you that a blockage or stagnation has released and chi is able to flow again.

Many Point Work techniques are available. The study of *Tui Na,* the original Chinese acupressure-massage, offers a huge variety of finger, hand, arm, and elbow techniques. The intention of each technique is to restore the free flow of chi and blood. By applying light pressure on an acupoint or meridian, you're bringing more chi and blood to the acupoint, or pool of energy. This in turn enhances the flow of chi and blood when it's been blocked or static.

Point Work is the center of the acupressure session. Everything you've done to assess your horse, decide what needs attending to, zeroing in on a specific organ system, and selecting acupoints has all led to this moment. Now it's time to work with the acupoints.

Remember, you're using both of your hands during Point Work. The working hand is applying pressure on the acupoint and the other hand is resting comfortably on the horse. The non-working hand acts as grounding and can help you feel for a reaction your horse might have.

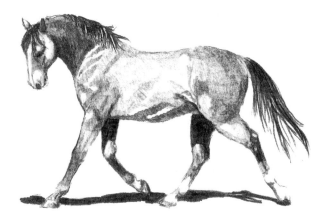

Thumb Technique

The thumb technique is used most frequently. It entails using the soft, fleshy portion of the tip of your thumb at a 45° to 90° angle to the horse's body. Apply light pressure initially because the meridian is just beneath the skin and horses are quite sensitive. As you're staying on the point, you can add a little pressure to encourage the movement of chi and blood.

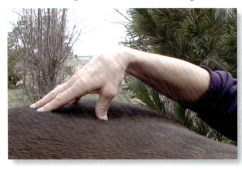

Thumb Technique: Place the soft tip of your thumb on the acupoint at a 45° to 90° angle to the horse's body or limb. Apply gentle pressure and place your non-working hand comfortably on the horse.

Two-Finger Technique

Take your middle finger and place it on top of the nail of your pointer finger to form a little tent. The point work is done with the soft tip of the pointer finger at a 45° to 90° angle from the horse's body. Whenever it becomes difficult to use the Thumb Technique, switch to the Two-Finger Technique. This technique tends to be used on the extremities.

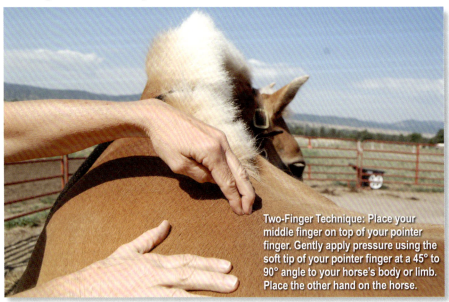

Two-Finger Technique: Place your middle finger on top of your pointer finger. Gently apply pressure using the soft tip of your pointer finger at a 45° to 90° angle to your horse's body or limb. Place the other hand on the horse.

Two-Finger Technique: Place your middle finger on top of your pointer finger. Gently apply pressure using the soft tip of your pointer finger at a 45° to 90° angle to your horse's body or limb. Place the other hand on the horse.

Because the meridians and acupoints are just beneath the surface of the skin, there is no need to press heavily or deeply. Instead, touch the point lightly because you don't know if any greater pressure would be painful. Point Work technique is best described by following the concept projected in "Muddy Water," which is included on the following page of this text.

The length of time you stay on an acupoint can vary. As a beginner, we suggest keeping your thumb on an acupoint for a very slow count of 1 to 30, while feeling for any changes in the point and observing your horse. If your horse gives any indication of discomfort with the pressure you're applying to an acupoint, move on to the next point or discontinue the session. There's no reason for your horse to be uncomfortable during an acupressure session.

The amount of time holding a point varies. When you are learning using the counting to 30 slowly technique is good. As your fingers become more educated, you'll feel the flow of chi beneath the skin and know when to go to the next acupoint. An acupoint can feel different ways, and as you're "working" it, you may feel a shift in the energy. Sometimes it's as simple as feeling a cool point warming or a warm point cooling or a hard point softening. Once the acupoint has shifted, it's time to move on.

Releases

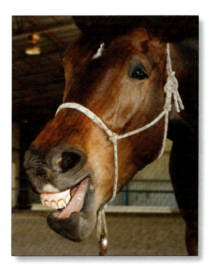

While you're holding an acupoint, the horse often gives you signs that energy is moving in his body. We call these "releases" due to the stimulation of acupoints. Releases are the horse's reactions to the chi moving again as well as his body assisting in promoting the flow of chi. Releases include: yawning, stretching, shaking, licking, passing air, rolling over, and sometimes even going to sleep!

Muddy Water
...the concept of Point Work Technique

The smooth-surfaced pond is clear and quiet, not even the smallest, softest ripple sullies the water.

If you were to plunge your hand into the pond and forcefully poke into the silt-layered bottom, spirals of tiny particles would rush up into the currents of water your hand created, disturbing the pool and obscuring your view and sense of what is beneath. By creating muddy water you would lose the ability to feel and know what really lays below that needs your attention.

But, when you gently cut the surface of this motionless pond and gently glide down to the bottom, the silt layers are revealed. You can feel and see what is there without creating a blinding torrent of silt and mud.

Kind, light touch on the first layer of silt bottom lets you know if there is pain. Come up a bit away to allow the slight drifting silt to settle back.

The first layer will give way to the second – rest the tip of your thumb momentarily on that place, what do you feel?

Is there a sense of energy in that place?
Is it dull, empty, cool, depressed?
Or, is it hot, protruding, angry?

It could be calm, mild, and smooth to the touch.

Come away from the point ever so slightly for a second, then return and gently be admitted to the third layer of silt, be content to stay there, not pressing, just hold that space.

Energy has its own pace, we are here to encourage, not force, not rush.

Hold that point with healing intention and wait for any resistance barrier to give way, stay the course, the resistance will pass and you will be meeting the need for energy to **break free and flow harmoniously.**

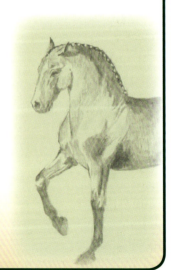

When you see and feel the horse releasing, stop holding the point and allow the natural process to continue and run its course. Then, go on to the next acupoint, or if the horse indicates he's done with the session, go ahead and perform the Closing described in the next section.

Closing

The last phase of the acupressure session is the Closing. It's a way of reconnecting the energy of the horse's body and tidying up any loose ends. The intention is to have a definite end to the session and leave your horse with a complete gift of acupressure.

Perform the Closing in exactly the way you began the session by repeating the Opening. By tracing the Bladder meridian with the heel of your hand three times on both sides of the horse you are again connecting with all the internal organs by virtue of the Association points. The difference is your *intention:* You're finishing and closing the energy.

You can vary the speed of tracing the Bladder meridian from head to hind coronary band, depending on how you want to leave the horse. If you want your horse to be calm and relaxed, trace the meridian slowly. If you think your horse needs an energy boost, trace the meridian more quickly in a fast sweep.

Post-Session

After the acupressure session, it's important to observe your horse's behavior and watch for any changes in the indicators that were apparent during your original assessment. It takes 24 hours for chi to flow throughout the meridian system, so you may not see observable changes during the first hours after a session. After the first 24 hours, make special note of any changes. By recording any changes, you will know what effect your session had on your horse.

The first 24 hours after a session is the time when chi is rebalancing. The second 24-hour period is when the horse's body is experiencing and adjusting to the shift in energy. On the third day, the effect of the session is seen more readily. This is why we often suggest people wait three days before offering another acupressure session. However, in specific situations, such as an in an emergency, you can do certain acupoints while waiting for the veterinarian to arrive and not a complete session.

Once you've contacted your holistic veterinarian, you can safely offer your horse specific acupoints in emergency situations, such as when he's experiencing colic, unconsciousness, or heatstroke, directly after surgery, before or after competition to calm him, and before training to focus him. You don't have to perform a complete session when you can help the horse right on the spot. Make this judgment call at the time by assessing the horse's needs.

Although a lot of theory and preparation related to acupressure seems complex, realize that acupressure works no matter how much or how little theory you know. The acupoints are doing what they do because of their inherent energetic characteristics and functions. A novice can perform a session that resolves the presenting health issue. The purpose of this book is to guide you through a comprehensive acupressure session.

…Seek veterinary care if there's even the slightest thought that the horse should be seen by a vet, please be sure to call.

Chapter Eleven

EQUINE SPECIFIC CONDITIONS

When you're learning how to cook, it helps to rely on "tried and true" recipes. Learning acupressure is similar. This chapter provides acupoint selection "recipes" for common equine physical and emotional conditions.

Centuries of clinical observation by highly trained Traditional Chinese Medicine doctors brings us a treasure trove of the energetic functions of acupoints. Why not start by working with acupoints known to have energetic attributes intended to resolve a specific condition?

The acupoints selected for each session have been proven to address these specific conditions. Using these points is a place to begin working with your horse once you've performed the assessment process discussed in Chapters Nine and Ten.

Take a few minutes to review the Four Examinations and the functions of the *zang-fu* organ systems. Addressing your horse's current condition is essential. And if you feel confident in your assessment, use the Association and Source points that are most directly applicable to the organ system related to your horse's pattern of disharmony.

For example, let's say Big Black's coat is looking flat and dusty. Just last week, it was as shiny as can be. When you touch his coat, it feels dry and the dust comes off on your hand. Which organ system supports the health of the coat? Lung controls skin and coat by dispersing chi. To select acupoints for a session, you can go back to the basic point selection technique given in Chapter Ten. To balance the Lung meridian, select Bladder 13 (Bl 13), the Association point for Lung, and Lung 9 (Lu 9), the Source point for Lung. This is a powerful set of four acupoints for your Point Work segment of your session, with the intention of resolving a Lung imbalance.

Ideally, you'll become proficient at working with the Association and Source points based on the energetics and functions of the *zang-fu* organs.

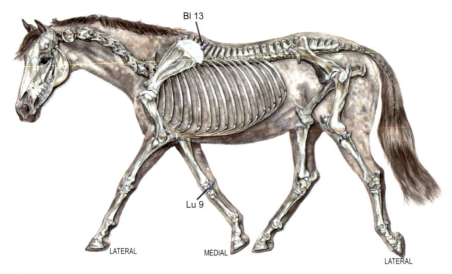

Acupoint selection for a Lung imbalance. Bladder 13 (Bl 13), Association point for Lung and Lung 9 (Lu 9), Source point for Lung, to be palpated on both sides of the horse.

It's just a matter of learning and practicing acupressure. Your sessions will have greater effectiveness as you progress.

The common condition charts in this chapter help you learn more about the functions and energetics of acupoints. This "cookbook" approach can yield a highly effective session, especially when you've carefully assessed your horse's condition. Having specific condition acupoints readily available offers you immediate access to the rich resources of Chinese medicine.

Remember, chi takes 24 hours to circulate throughout the body. You may not see any change during the first 24-hour cycle. In fact, your horse may seem worse. This is not uncommon, the animal can appear to be sicker than before, which is known as a healing crisis. What's actually happening is that the "illness" is moving through his body and is being resolved. Of course, if your horse's condition continues to deteriorate, consult your veterinarian.

Observe your horse for the next two to three days to detect changes. If your horse is receiving the therapeutic effect you intended, include these same acupoints in your next session. If there's little or no benefit, vary your acupoints based on the organ systems involved or other points suggested in this chapter.

Local and Distal Acupoints

Once you know the location of the 12 Major Meridians and two Extraordinary Vessels, you're able to work with another method of selecting acupoints. That is, you can use the acupoints in the vicinity of where the actual problem is located. This is called using local points for musculoskeletal issues and specific organ imbalances.

For example, Dandy has been lame on his off-side foreleg. Your vet tells you that Dandy has a minor tendon injury located on the medial aspect (inside) of his leg. You can use acupoints above and below the painful area on his leg where specific meridians are passing through the injured area. The Lung, Pericardium, and Heart meridians flow along the medial side of the horse's forelimb. This technique helps move both chi and blood through the injury.

Using local acupoints is often combined with selecting a "distal" point. A distal acupoint has the energetics affecting the area or issue related to the injury. Gall Bladder 34 (GB 34) is considered a distal point for Dandy's tendon injury. GB 34 is located on the hind limb—a *distance* from the injury site—and has the effect of enhancing the supply of nourishment to his tendons.

Another example of how to use local and distal acupoints is when your horse has conjunctivitis (inflammation of the mucous membrane that lines the exposed portion of the eyeball and inner surface of the eyelids). The local points surrounding the eye are: Bladder 1, Stomach 2, and Gall Bladder 1. The distal point you can include in your point selection is Liver 2, located on the hind leg. Liver 2 is known to benefit the health and sensory acuity of the eye.

Distal points can come into play when your horse is hypersensitive or has sustained an injury that's particularly painful. Better to stay away from the offending location and use acupoints that will benefit the problem and are at a distance.

You don't have to use all of the points on the charts in one session; use only two or three points for your first acupressure session. If those acupoints yield the effect you intend, repeat them in the second session. If not, use other suggested acupoints.

The acupoints given for specific equine conditions in the following pages are general points. The points presented may not address the exact moment in the progression of your horse's current problem nor the root of your horse's health issue. Remember to record your assessment, point selections, observations, and any significant reactions your horse has to the acupressure session for the following 24- to 48-hours post-session.

Because you have to start somewhere, start where you're comfortable and think you can benefit your horse most. It takes study, understanding, and practice to become proficient at selecting acupoints that address your horse's health and behavior conditions. The key is to start!

Horses change lives. They give our young people confidence and self-esteem. They provide peace and tranquility to troubled souls, they give us hope."

— Toni Robinson

EQUINE AGING

In Chinese Medicine, aging is the natural process directly related to Kidney function. The Essence chi, or jing, of the horse is housed in the Kidney. The foal arrives on earth with a certain amount of Essence chi depending on the health and conformation of the dam and sire. This Essence chi diminishes as the animal grows to maturity and old age. When there's no longer enough Essence chi to sustain the horse's life he dies.

The horse's *zang-fu* organ system function slows during his declining years. His musculoskeletal strength and vitality diminish. These anatomical and emotional (*shen*) changes are indicative of a loss of Essence chi. The General Aging acupressure session provided in this section offers a way to help support your horse during his later years.

It's very common for older horses to develop degenerative osteoarthritis. And, it's the most common equine joint disease. Arthritis is not limited to aging horses, younger horses can experience osteoarthritis, too. It can be the result of impact trauma, injury, over-use, infection, poor conformation, hereditary issues, mineral or dietary deficiencies, as well as aging. Horses involved in competitive activities are more apt to develop arthritis at an earlier age due to the increased stress on their joints.

Being aware of common causes combined with early detection of arthritis affords you the opportunity to slow the progression of the disease. Early signs of arthritis include:

- Mild swelling and heat in the joint
- Reluctance or refusal to perform in his usual sport
- Stiffness following inactivity
- Decrease in joint flexibility (range of motion)
- Crunching ("crepitus") sound when the joint is flexed
- Tenderness of joint upon palpation
- Tiring more quickly than usual
- Sudden attitude or mood change

As the condition progresses, these indicators become more exaggerated, plus – your horse will most likely exhibit some degree of lameness because his joints are painful. Arthritis hurts.

General Aging

Indicators
- Overall slowing down
- Loss of strength and muscle tone
- Increased need for rest
- Decreased interest in training

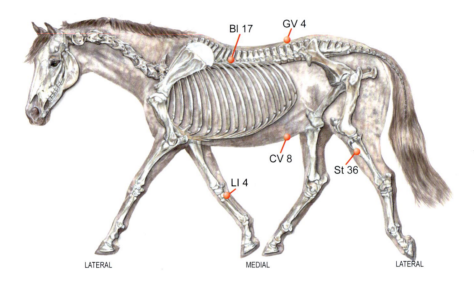

Point	Name	Location
LI 4	Adjoining Valley	Found distal and medial to the head of the medial splint bone.
St 36	Leg 3 Miles	One half (0.5) cun lateral to the tibial crest, on the lateral side of the tibia.
Bl 17	Diaphragm's Transport	Three cun lateral to the dorsal midline in the 12th intercostal space.
CV 8	Spirit's Palace Gate	Found in the center of the umbilicus.
GV 4	Vital Gate	On the dorsal midline in depression between lumbar vertebrae 2 and 3.

OSTEOARTHRITIS

By the age of fifteen, the horse's body produces cartilage at a slower rate than it is being worn away. The synovial fluid, which lubricates the joints and helps the joint glide, tends to become thin and less plentiful with age.

When cartilage is worn away and there's less synovial fluid in the joint, the opposing bones receive greater impact. As a horse ages, (or a young horse due to other factors such as injury), his tendons and ligaments are not as strong and flexible as they need to be for joint stability. These conditions can lead to joint instability, inflammation, pronounced swelling and obvious lameness. The body's natural reaction to this painful condition is to grow more bone in an attempt to protect itself. The over-growth of bone engenders severe osteoarthritis. This condition is very painful and mobility is compromised.

In TCM, osteoarthritis is considered a type of "Bi Syndrome," which is a painful condition characterized by a blockage of chi and blood circulation. More specifically, osteoarthritis is called a "Bony Bi Pattern of Disharmony." This pattern is brought about by an invasion of external pathogens such as Wind, Cold, Damp and Heat. In general, arthritis is a deficiency pattern.

Selection of acupoints for osteoarthritis depends on how and where this degenerative joint disease manifests. Commonly, arthritis presents in the following four conditions:

- Joints Exhibit Heat
- Migrating Pain
- Worse with Cold Weather
- Worse with Wet Weather

Assess how your horse is experiencing arthritis and choose acupoints from the chart most applicable to his condition. We all want our horses to enjoy active lives for as long as possible.

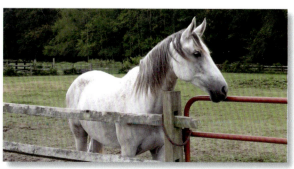

Joints Exhibit Heat

There's an acute inflammation of the joint tissues. However, the underlying condition is actually a chronic cold condition due to the degeneration of cartilage and bone. The painful rubbing of bone on bone leads to the inflammation of the tissues in and surrounding the joint.

Indicators

- Acutely painful (sudden onset)
- Joints are swollen and hot
- Pain increases with pressure
- Minimal mobility

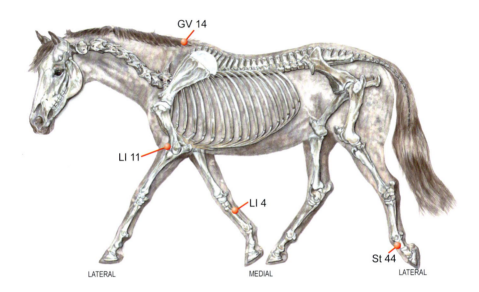

Point	Name	Location
LI 4	Adjoining Valley	Found distal and medial to the head of the medial splint bone.
LI 11	Crooked Pool	On the lateral aspect of the foreleg in a depression cranial to the elbow in the transverse cubital crease.
St 44	Inner Courtyard	Craniodistal to the fetlock, caudal to the long digital extensor muscle.
GV 14	Big Vertebra	On the dorsal midline in a depression between the 7th cervical and 1st thoracic vertebrae cranial to the highest point of the withers.

Migrating Pain

One day your mare seems to be favoring her nearside foreleg, the next day her offside hind is obviously stiff and painful. This is the nature of arthritic migrating pain.

Indicators

- Shifting lameness
- Reluctance to perform
- Lethargy

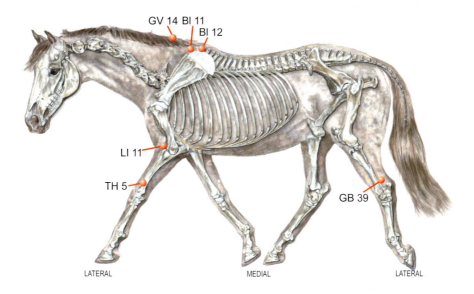

Point	Name	Location
LI 11	Crooked Pond	On the lateral aspect of the foreleg in a depression cranial to the elbow in the transverse cubital crease.
Bl 11	Great Shuttle	One and one half (1.5) cun lateral to dorsal midline at about the 3rd thoracic vertebra cranial to the withers.
Bl 12	Wind's Gate	At the highest point of withers at about the 4th thoracic vertebral space.
TH 5	Outer Gate	Between the radius and ulna 2 cun above TH 4. Opposite Pe 6.
GB 39	Suspended Bell	Three cun above the tip of the lateral malleolus in a depression on the caudal aspect of the tibia.
GV 14	Big Vertebra	On the dorsal midline in a depression between the 7th cervical and 1st thoracic vertebrae cranial to the highest point of the withers.

Worse in Cold Weather

Indicators
- Debilitating pain or deep ache
- Tissues surrounding the joint may be involved
- Arthritic area may feel cold
- Cold increases pain

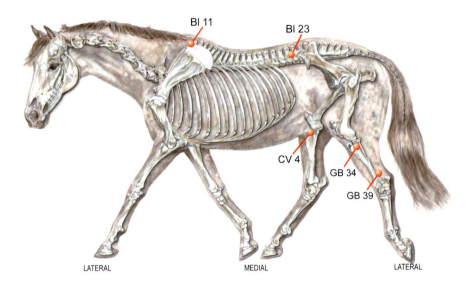

Point	Name	Location
Bl 11	Great Shuttle	One and one half (1.5) cun lateral to dorsal midline at about the 3rd thoracic vertebra cranial to the withers.
Bl 23	Kidney's Transport	Three cun lateral to the dorsal midline between the 2nd and 3rd lumbar vertebrae directly dorsal to the ventral end of the last rib.
GB 34	Yang Mound Spring	In the interosseous space between the tibia and fibula between the long and lateral digital extensors, craniodistal to the head of the fibula.
GB 39	Suspended Bell	Three cun above the tip of the lateral malleolus in a depression on the caudal aspect of the tibia.
CV 4	Gate to Original Chi	On the ventral midline 3 cun caudal to the umbilicus.

Worse in Wet Weather

Indicators

- Joints are stiff and/or ache
- Damp-cold environment increases discomfort
- Possible edema of the joints and lower leg

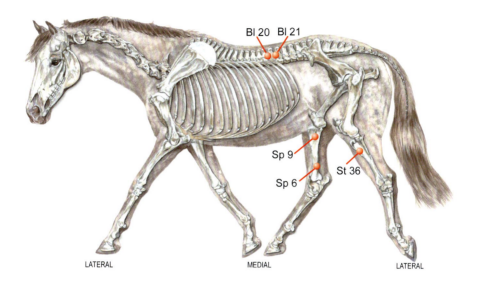

Point	Name	Location
St 36	Leg 3 Miles	One half (0.5) cun lateral to the tibial crest on the lateral side of the tibia.
Sp 6	3 Yin Meeting	Three cun above the tip of the medial malleolus, caudal to the tibial border on the medial aspect of hind leg. 0.5 cun posterior to the saphenous vein of the hindlimb.
Sp 9	Yin Mound Spring	In a depression at the level of the patellar ligaments 0.5 cun in front of the saphenous vein.
Bl 20	Spleen's Transport	Three cun lateral to the dorsal midline in the last (17th) intercostal space.
Bl 21	Stomach's Transport	Three cun lateral to the dorsal midline caudal to the last rib.

BEHAVIOR ISSUES

Before assuming your horse has a behavior issue, be sure to check him out yourself and have your holistic veterinarian out to see him. Equine behavior issues are often physical or equipment problems. If she is hurting, she is not going to be cooperative. And, if she is not able to do something she did easily last week, there may be a good reason.

Remember, horses do their best to appear sound and keep up with the herd even when they are in pain. In the wild, the herd will leave them behind with no protection when they give signs of physical weakness. A sick or injured horse threatens the safety of the herd. Horses are hardwired to not show pain until its completely debilitating. A change in behavior is often the first indicator of discomfort or pain.

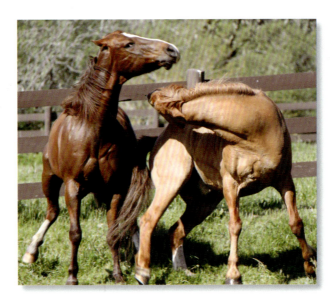

Once you've ruled out a physical issue or discomfort from equipment as the reason for the undesirable behavior your horse is exhibiting, it's time to look at possible environmental factors. There are numerous reasons a horse has a behavior issue such as incompatible training style, herd management issues, and other stressors your horse may be experiencing.

Simply by virtue of the horse's inherent nature as a flight-versus-fight animal coupled with domestication of the species leaves us with an animal bound to have a variety of behavior issues. Their willingness to let us be "boss mare" fits with their natural hierarchical herd behavior. But, having a human on their back is not natural and being "broken" can be nasty business for a horse.

Somehow horses have adapted to our insistence they live in small spaces, eat what we give them, and perform in work and sport as we demand. Their pliant nature is remarkable. However, there are limits. Horses are sentient beings with feelings and their own physical and emotional needs. When they are overly stressed they have to express it in some manner that may not be particularly pleasant for us. They may even evince their stress in a way that's harmful to themselves, which is even more distressing.

Cribbing, anhidrosis, and anxiety have a strong component related to stress which cause physical harm. We have to be careful not to confuse the horses' docile nature with their experience of what we expect of them and how we manage their care. There are many equine behaviorist who can give you insights into your horse's behavior, we will leave that to them.

If you are reading and working with *ACU-HORSE: A Guide to Equine Acupressure* the odds are you're making an effort to work in partnership with your horse. Luckily, you know that the "master-slave" model of equine training and management creates a highly stressful experience for all concerned. Even with a more natural, harmonious, and thoughtful approach to working with your horse, including acupressure routines in your care and tending will contribute to your horse's health and well-being.

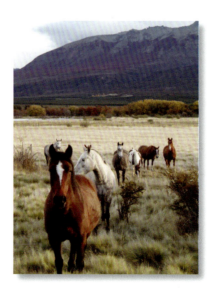

CRIBBING

Cribbing is also called crib biting or windsucking. It's considered a compulsive stable vice where a horse bites the stable door or fencing, arches his neck, and sucks in air. There seems to be a connection to the horse's response to confinement, possible dietary issues, colic, and ulcers. Cribbing releases natural endorphins which is calming and thought to reduce stress and discomfort.

There's evidence that grain-fed horses crib to neutralize stomach acid. The increased saliva produced by cribbing can help reduce stomach acid, a by-product of feeding grain. Horses with stomach ulcers may resort to cribbing to neutralize stomach acid.

Indicators

- Agitation when confined
- Digestive issues
- Stomach ulcers
- Acidic stomach fluids
- Colic
- Cribbing behavior

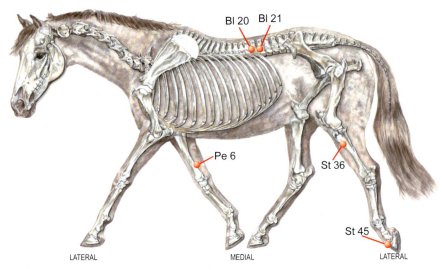

Point	Name	Location
St 36	Leg 3 Miles	One half (0.5) cun lateral to the tibial crest on the lateral side of the tibia.
St 45	Evil's Dissipation	Located just lateral to the cranial midline of the hind hoof, proximal to the coronary band.
Bl 20	Spleen's Transport	Three cun lateral to dorsal midline in the last (17th) intercostal space.
Bl 21	Stomach's Transport	Three cun lateral to dorsal midline caudal to last rib.
Pe 6	Inner Gate	Located on medial aspect of foreleg, about 2 cun above Pe 7, directly cranial to mid-point of chestnut.

FEAR

As a prey animal, fear is a successful survival strategy. A horse with no fear is a dangerous animal both to himself and you. And, too much fear can be equally dangerous for the horse and you. Your horse's flight instinct is absolutely normal. Helping him stay within reasonable limits is a good idea. The following acupressure session can help when your horse tends to give into his fears more than not or has less fear than seems healthy. The intent is to balance his emotional reactions.

Indicators

- Increased flight response
- Resistance to training
- Insecurity
- Rearing frequently
- Abnormal response to change
- Heightened response to a specific trigger
- Anxiety around fearful people
- Confusion in communication

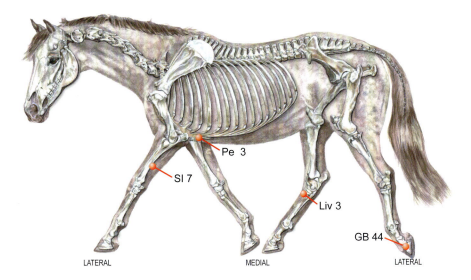

Point	Name	Location
SI 7	Branch to Heart	On the caudolateral aspect of forelimb about 6 cun above SI 5.
Pe 3	Marsh at the Crook	On the medial side of the cubital crease of the elbow cranial to Heart 3.
Liv 3	Great Thoroughfare	On the craniomedial aspect of the cannon bone at the level of the head of the medial splint bone.
GB 44	Foot Yin's Aperture	On the craniolateral aspect of the coronary band on the hind limb.

Focus for Training

Indicators

- Easily distracted
- Resistance to training
- Short attention span
- Restlessness
- Irritability

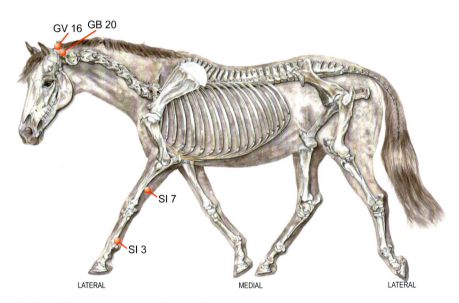

Point	Name	Location
SI 3	Back Stream	In a depression on the distal end of the lateral splint bone on the caudolateral border of the cannon bone.
SI 7	Branch to Heart	On the caudolateral aspect of forelimb about 6 cun above SI 5.
GB 20	Wind Pool	In the large depression caudal to the occipital condyle.
GV 16	Wind's Palace	On the dorsal midline in a depression between the occipital protuberances, at the atlantooccipital joint.

GRIEF

Indicators
- Lethargic disposition
- Dull eye
- No interest in activity
- Depressed nature

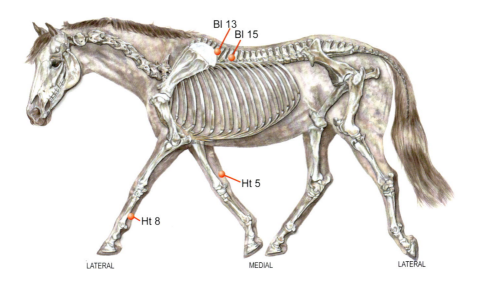

Point	Name	Location
Ht 5	Communication's Route	On the caudal aspect of the radius in depression at about the level of the accessory carpal bone.
Ht 8	Lesser Palace	On the caudolateral aspect of 3rd metacarpal bone cranial to the deep flexor tendon.
Bl 13	Lung's Transport	Three cun lateral to the dorsal midline in the 8th intercostal space.
Bl 15	Heart's Transport	Three cun lateral to the dorsal midline in the 10th intercostal space.

Nervousness / Anxiety

Indicators

- Compulsive behaviors (stable vices)
- Destructive behaviors
- Volatile emotional responses
- Loose manure
- Inappropriate sweating
- Self-mutilation
- Striking or biting inappropriately

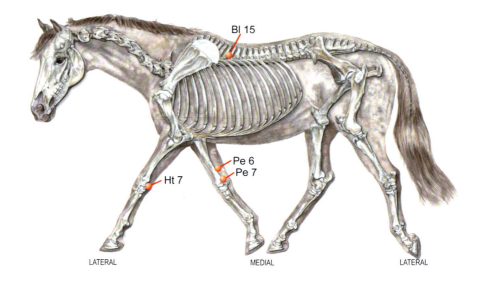

Point	Name	Location
Ht 7	Spirit's Gate	Caudolateral aspect of the radius, proximal to the accessory carpal bone. Opposite Pe 7.
Bl 15	Heart's Transport	Three cun lateral to the dorsal midline in the 10th intercostal space.
Pe 6	Inner Gate	Located on the medial aspect of the foreleg about 2 cun above Pe 7, directly cranial to the mid-point of the chestnut.
Pe 7	Big Mound	Found at the level of the accessory carpal bone on the medial aspect of the foreleg.

GASTROINTESTINAL ISSUES

Though the equine gastrointestinal tract provided an important evolutionary edge in their survival, this same digestive process poses some distinct disadvantages as all horse people know. The horse is designed to consume low-nutrient forage along with lots of water to smooth its passage throughout its route through the horse's body. Horses are well adapted to grass lands where they travel 20 or more miles a day to graze and satisfy their nutritional needs.

Now place the horse in a domesticated environment. They are at the mercy of whatever we think they should consume. This can include high fiber grasses and high potency grains along with supplements of all sorts. Not having sufficient body movement to maintain healthy motility can affect the digestive process as well. Just living in a domesticated environment creates stress with which their wild counterparts don't have to contend.

Frequency of feeding, quantity of fiber, sufficient turn out, and nutritional sufficiency can contribute to gastrointestinal problems. Horses are meant to graze with their necks extended downward so the saliva-infused bolus can travel up the esophagus as it begins the digestive process. When we feed from raised feeders we are disrupting that process. There are many natural equine resources available for you to arrive at what's best for your horse.

Unfortunately, even with the best care and intentions, your horse can experience digestive problems including ingesting toxic substances, infections, parasites, overeating, gastric ulcers, colic, etc. The acupressure sessions provided regarding the gastrointestinal tract are intended to help prevent digestive problems before they occur. If your horse has a tendency toward any of these difficulties, these routines can support his digestive health.

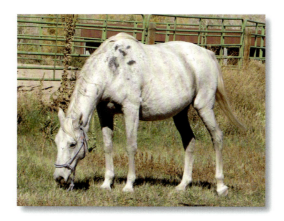

Flatulent Colic

Flatulent or gas colic is the most common form of colic. It is the result of the fermentation process during digestion forming abnormal bowel distention.

Indicators

- Abdominal bloating
- Gaseous gut sounds
- Kicking and/or biting at abdomen
- Indicators can be intermittent

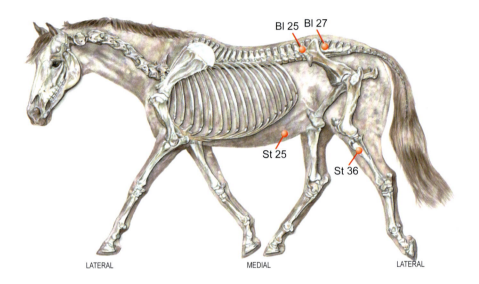

Point	Name	Location
St 25	Heaven's Axis	Located 2 cun lateral to the umbilicus.
St 36	Leg 3 Miles	One half cun lateral to the tibial crest on the lateral side of the tibia.
Bl 25	Large Intestine's Transport	Three cun lateral to the dorsal midline between the 5th and 6th lumbar vertebrae at the cranial edge of the wings of the ilium.
Bl 27	Small Intestine's Transport	Three cun lateral to the dorsal midline between the 1st and 2nd sacral vertebrae.

Impaction Colic

Impaction or obstructive colic is the most serious form of colic. This occurs when there's an accumulation of food substances in the bowel forming a blockage thus prohibiting movement of food through the large colon.

Indicators

- Consistent, severe pain
- Reluctance to eat
- Refusal to drink water
- Dehydration
- No gut sounds
- Elevated heart and respiration rates
- Incapacity to produce manure
- General colic indicators

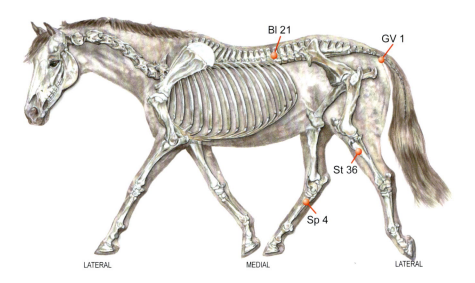

Point	Name	Location
St 36	Leg 3 Miles	One half (0.5) cun lateral to the tibial crest on the lateral side of the tibia.
Sp 4	Grandfather / Grandson	In a depression on the hind leg mediodistal to the head of the medial splint bone.
Bl 21	Stomach's Transport	Three cun lateral to the dorsal midline caudal to the last rib.
GV 1	Lasting Strength	On the dorsal midline in a depression between the anus and the base of the tail.

Prevention of Colic

When you know your horse has a tendency toward any form of colic, the following session can be offered every four or five days. Chinese medicine is best known for its capacity to prevent health issues.

Indicators

- Distended abdomen
- Abdominal pain
- Agitation or restlessness
- Kicking or biting flank
- Lying down
- Sweating
- Pawing at the ground
- Rolling on the ground
- Possible increased heart rate

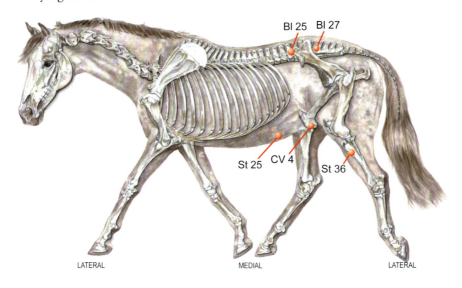

Point	Name	Location
St 25	Heaven's Axis	Located 2 cun lateral to the umbilicus.
St 36	Leg 3 Miles	One half (0.5) cun lateral to the tibial crest, on the lateral side of the tibia.
Bl 25	Large Intestine's Transport	Three cun lateral to the dorsal midline between the 5th and 6th lumbar vertebrae at the cranial edge of the wings of the ilium.
Bl 27	Small Intestine's Transport	Three cun lateral to the dorsal midline between the 1st and 2nd sacral vertebrae.
CV 4	Gate to Original Chi	On the ventral midline 3 cun caudal to the umbilicus.

IMPROVE DIGESTION

The following acupressure routine is intended for general digestion and to maintain balance along the gastrointestinal tract. It is a good session to support nutrient absorption and avoid possible imbalances that could disrupt the digestive process.

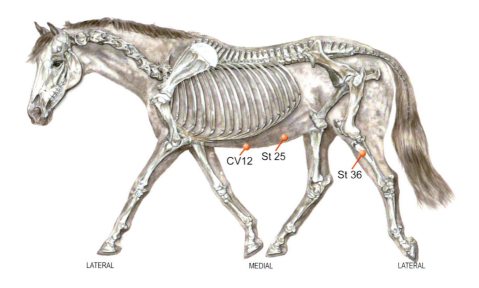

Point	Name	Location
St 25	Heaven's Axis	Located 2 cun lateral to the umbilicus.
St 36	Leg 3 Miles	One half cun lateral to the tibial crest on the lateral side of the tibia.
CV 12	Sea of Power	On the ventral midline halfway between the xiphoid process and the umbilicus.

Diarrhea / Constipation

The acupoints selected to help resolve diarrhea are the same as resolving constipation because these points are known to balance the gastrointestinal tract. By balancing the entire digestive system when there's either too much fluid or too little fluid in the manure, the issue can be resolved. In TCM, returning the body back to a harmonious flow of chi is the intent so the body can heal itself.

Indicators
- Loose, watery manure
- Dry, hard manure

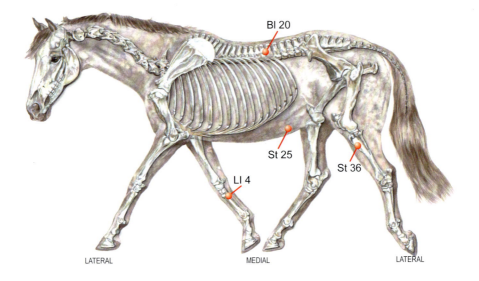

Point	Name	Location
LI 4	Adjoining Valley	Found distal and medial to the head of the medial splint bone.
St 25	Heaven's Axis	Located 2 cun lateral to the umbilicus.
St 36	Leg 3 Miles	One half (0.5) cun lateral to the tibial crest on the lateral side of the tibia.
Bl 20	Spleen's Transport	Three cun lateral to the dorsal midline in the last, (17th) intercostal space.

GENERAL CONDITIONS
Immune System Issues

Every horse on earth can benefit from strengthening his immune system every third or fourth day. Make it part of your grooming routine. Our horses are constantly exposed to environmental toxins, dust, pollens, and other potential allergens. It's a fact of modern life. If your horse has a strong immune system his body will be able to cope with whatever is in his environment. If his Defensive chi, *Wei* chi, is not strong, these allergens can invade his body and compromise his health.

In Chinese medicine, much of illness is attributed to not having a strong immune system. Hence, a strong immune system is the key to good health and longevity. The organ systems that most affect the immune system are Lung, Kidney, and Liver. The following acupoints are known to support these *zang-fu* organs:

- **Lung 7** – Stimulates the descending and dispersing of Lung chi and Defensive chi.
- **Large Intestine 4** – Tonifies chi flow and Defensive chi.
- **Stomach 36** – Strengthens the body by tonifying chi and blood.
- **Spleen 6** – Nourishes blood and yin chi, promotes Liver function.
- **Bladder 23** – Supports and nourishes Kidney chi and essence.
- **Governing Vessel 14** – Regulates Nutritive and Defensive chi.

The Immune System Strengthening acupressure session can be used as a general health maintenance session and to support your horse's healing after surgery, trauma, or vaccinations.

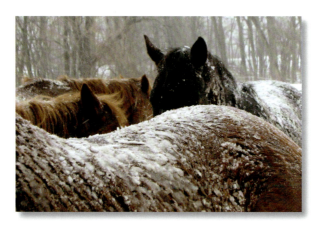

Immune System Strengthening

Indicators

- Exposure to toxins
- Vaccinosis
- Reaction to medication
- Exposure to infectious disease
- Slow healing of superficial wound
- Frequent or chronic infection or illness
- Exhibiting allergic reaction (skin irritation, nasal or eye discharge)

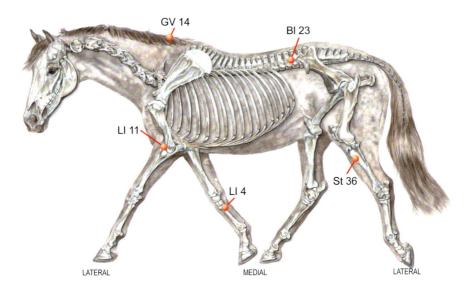

Point	Name	Location
LI 4	Adjoining Valley	Found distal and medial to the head of the medial splint bone.
LI 11	Crooked Pond	On the lateral aspect of the foreleg in a depression cranial to the elbow in the transverse cubital crease.
St 36	Leg 3 Miles	One half (0.5) cun lateral to the tibial crest on the lateral side of the tibia.
Bl 23	Kidney's Transport	Three cun lateral to the dorsal midline between the 2nd and 3rd lumbar vertebrae directly dorsal to the ventral end of the last rib.
GV 14	Big Vertebra	On the dorsal midline in a depression between the 7th cervical and 1st thoracic vertebrae cranial to the highest point of the withers.

Edema

A swelling caused by fluid in body tissue is called an edema. Localized edemas tend to form in the lower extremities, ventral midline on a horse's trunk, and on the face. Generalized edema is usually first seen as swelling of the horses facial region. An edema is often due to confinement, thyroid issue, reaction to bug bites, or exposure to toxins. Have your holistic veterinarian check your horse if he's exhibiting an edema.

Indicators

- Facial swelling
- Swelling of the legs
- Swelling along the ventral midline

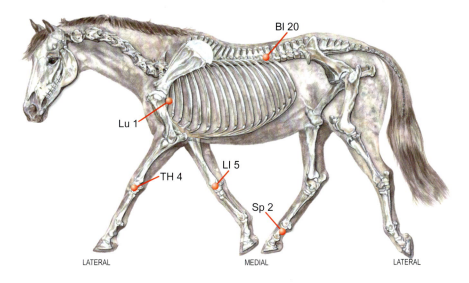

Point	Name	Location
Lu 1	Central Palace	Located in the depression in the center of the muscle belly of the descending pectoral muscle at the level of the 1st intercostal space.
LI 5	Yang Stream	In a depression between the 2nd and 3rd carpal bones on the craniomedial aspect of the carpus.
Sp 2	Great Metropolis	Distal to the medial sesamoid bone at the caudal border of the tendon.
Bl 20	Spleen's Transport	Three cun lateral to the dorsal midline in the last (17th) intercostal space.
TH 4	Yang's Pool	In a large depression slightly lateral to the middle of the cranial surface of the carpal joint between the intermediate and 3rd carpal bones.

HOOF PROBLEM / Founder (Laminitis)

Founder is a common hoof condition involving the inflammation and degeneration of the laminae (white line), the tissue connecting the pedal bone to the hoof.

Founder is thought to be a metabolic imbalance which restricts blood flow to the hoof resulting in the inner hoof capsule tearing away from the hoof wall. This leads to the rotation or sinking of the coffin bone because it's no longer supported in the hoof capsule. At its extreme the coffin bone can penetrate through the sole.

There are many causes identified such as carbohydrate overload, a serious colic event, nitrogen compound overload, untreated infection, sudden change in diet, insulin resistance, rich pasture grass, trauma to the sole, poor circulation, excessive weight…to mention a few.

Indicators
- Lameness
- Obvious pain standing
- Stretched white line
- Leaning back stance / Lying down
- Short gait with tentative foot placement
- Continuously shifting weight
- X-ray imaging

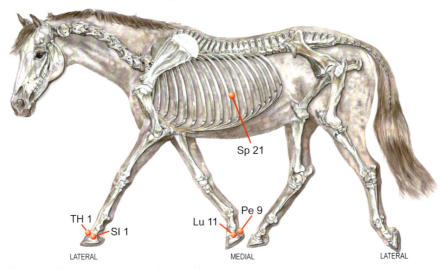

Point	Name	Location
Lu 11	Lesser Metal's Note	Caudomedial aspect of forelimb at coronary band.
Sp 21	General Control	At level of shoulder joint in the 10th intercostal space.
SI 1	Young Marsh	On craniolateral aspect of front hoof at coronary band.
Pe 9	Middle Rushing	At the center of the depression between the heel bulbs on the forelimb.
TH 1	Gate's Rushing	Just lateral to the cranial midline of the front hoof proximal to the coronary band.

MUSCULOSKELETAL ISSUES

The term "musculoskeletal" pertains to the system containing the striated muscles (not the smooth or cardiac muscles) and the bony skeleton. Issues related to the musculoskeletal system are often considered Bi Syndromes in TCM. Bi Syndromes are characterized by stiffness and pain attributed to the stagnation or blockage of blood and chi within the horse's meridian system.

In TCM, this type of pain is linked to an invasion of external pathogens such as Wind, Cold, Damp, Heat, or Dryness. Sometimes the root of the obstruction of blood and chi are a combination of these pathogens. For instance, the body tends to constrict when invaded by Wind-Cold. These pathogens cut off the supply of chi and blood to part of the horse's body, like the shoulder or neck…thus constricting that area.

Although musculoskeletal issues are more common for older horses, younger horses can exhibit clinical signs of muscle-bone issues due to illness, injury, surgical procedures, poor breeding, and poor quality food.

Remember, your holistic veterinarian is your best resource for trauma care, if your horse is in extreme pain or any prolonged indications of movement issues. Acupressure is best suited to working with the prevention of musculoskeletal problems and available to manage any issues after you have followed your veterinarian's recommendations.

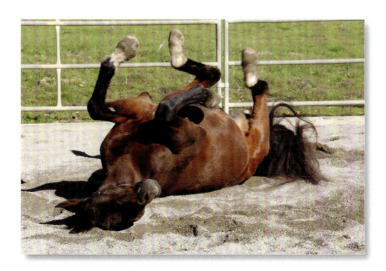

Cervical / Neck Issues

Indicators
- Restricted or painful neck movement
- Unusual or inappropriate head carriage
- Difficulty raising or lowering the head
- Elevated heart rate
- Resistance to movement
- Lameness
- Agitation
- Swelling or bruising

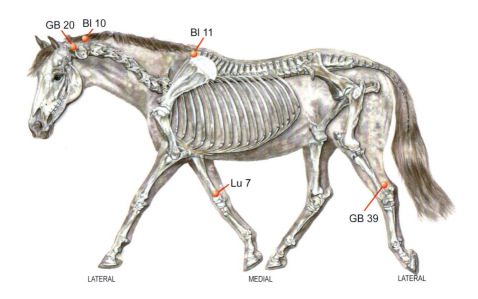

Point	Name	Location
Lu 7	Broken Sequence	Located just cranial to the cephalic vein at the level of the distal border of the chestnut.
Bl 10	Heaven's Pillar	Two cun off the dorsal midline in a depression caudal to the wings of the atlas.
Bl 11	Great Shuttle	One and one-half (1.5) cun lateral to dorsal midline at about the 3rd thoracic vertebra cranial to the withers.
GB 20	Wind Pool	In the large depression caudal to the occipital condyle.
GB 39	Suspended Bell	Three cun above the tip of the lateral malleolus in a depression on the caudal aspect of the tibia.

Hock Issues

Indicators
- Lameness
- Lack of hind leg impulsion
- Swelling or heat around joint
- Shifting weight
- Reluctance to train

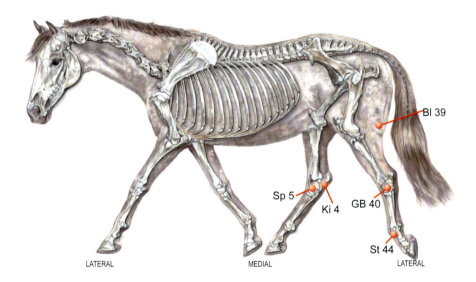

Point	Name	Location
St 44	Inner Courtyard	Craniodistal to the fetlock, caudal to the long digital extensor muscle.
Sp 5	Metal's Note Hill	In a depression cranial and distal to the medial malleolus, on the saphenous vein.
Bl 39	Entrusting Yang	At the ventral edge of the muscle groove at the level of the stifle cranial to Bl 40.
Ki 4	Big Bell	Found 0.5 cun caudodistal to Ki 3 on the medial border of the Achilles tendon.
GB 40	Hill's Ruins	Found craniodistal to the tip of lateral malleolus of the tibia over the tendon of the lateral digital extensor.

Lower Back Soreness

Indicators
- Resistance to tacking up or grooming
- Unable to move comfortably
- Difficulty changing gaits
- Uneven gait
- Restlessness or irritability
- Swelling or heat along dorsal midline

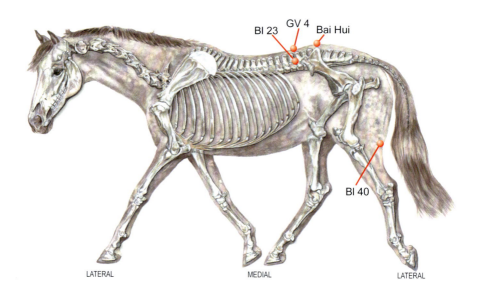

Point	Name	Location
Bl 23	Kidney's Transport	Three cun lateral to the dorsal midline between the 2nd and 3rd lumbar vertebrae directly dorsal to the ventral end of the last rib.
Bl 40	Supporting the Middle	At the midpoint of the transverse crease of the popliteal fossa.
Bai Hui	100 Meetings	On the dorsal midline at the lumbosacral space.
GV 4	Vital Gate	On the dorsal midline in a depression between lumbar vertebrae 2 and 3.

PRE-PERFORMANCE

Anywhere from one to three hours prior to any type of performance, including an easy trail ride or a strenuous endurance ride, it's wise to offer your horse this Pre-Performance Acupressure routine. It will aid in bringing nourishment to all of your horse's soft and bony tissues by enhancing the circulation of chi and blood. The outcome of this routine is supple tendons and ligaments, muscles at the ready, and resilient, strong bones. It's so important for the horse to have a well-nourished body so he can perform optimally and without injury.

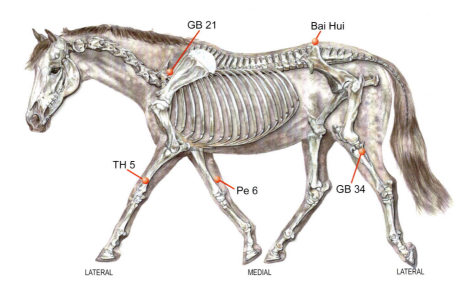

Point	Name	Location
Pe 6	Inner Gate	Located on the medial aspect of the foreleg about 2 cun above Pe 7, directly cranial to the mid-point of the chestnut.
TH 5	Outer Gate	Found between the radius and ulna 2 cun above TH 4. Opposite Pe 6.
GB 21	Shoulder Well	At the midpoint of the cranial edge of the scapula.
GB 34	Yang Mound Spring	In the interosseous space between the tibia and fibula between the long and lateral digital extensors, craniodistal to the head of the fibula.
Bai Hui	100 Meetings	On the dorsal midline at the lumbosacral space.

Post-Performance

The best time to give your horse a Post-Performance acupressure routine is right after your horse has cooled down. The acupoints used in the acupressure session will help supply your horse's body with nutrients while also removing the harmful buildup of toxins in his soft tissues. It's a good way for your horse to recover from activity and strengthen his muscles, tendons, and bones.

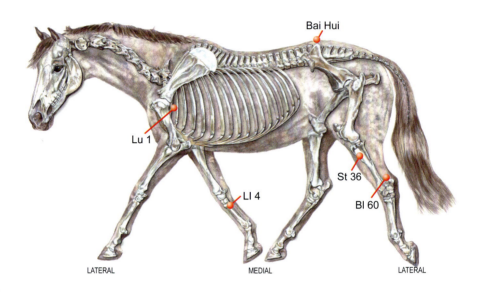

Point	Name	Location
Lu 1	Central Palace	Located in the depression in the center of the muscle belly of the descending pectoral muscle at the level of the 1st intercostal space.
LI 4	Adjoining Valley	Found distal and medial to the head of the medial splint bone.
St 36	Leg 3 Miles	One half (0.5) cun lateral to the tibial crest on the lateral side of the tibia.
Bl 60	Kunlun Mountain	Between the lateral malleolus of the tibia and the calcaneal tuber. Opposite Ki 3.
Bai Hui	100 Meetings	On the dorsal midline at the lumbosacral space.

Shoulder Soreness

Indicators

- Forelimb lameness
- Difficulty changing directions or turning
- Difficulty in slowing down or stopping
- Difficulty in going up or down hills
- Trouble getting up or down
- Resistance to movement
- Excessive lying down

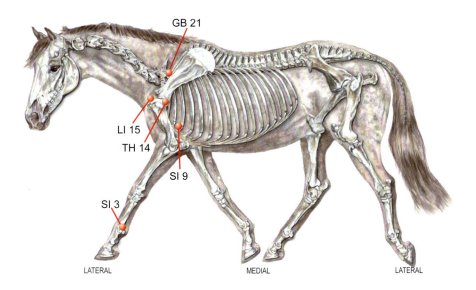

Point	Name	Location
LI 15	Shoulder's Corner	Found just cranial to the point of shoulder.
SI 3	Back Stream	In depression on distal end of the lateral splint bone on the caudolateral border of the cannon bone.
SI 9	Upright Shoulder	In a depression at the caudal border of the deltoid muscle where it meets the lateral and long heads of the triceps brachii.
TH 14	Shoulder Opening	On the caudal edge of shoulder joint, at the level of the point of shoulder.
GB 21	Shoulder Well	Found at the midpoint of the cranial edge of the scapula.

Stifle Issues

Indicators
- Hind limb lameness
- Reluctance to change gaits
- Lack of hind leg impulsion
- Swelling or heat around joint
- Difficulty changing directions or turning
- Difficulty in slowing down or stopping
- Difficulty in going up or down hills
- Trouble getting up or down
- Resistance to movement

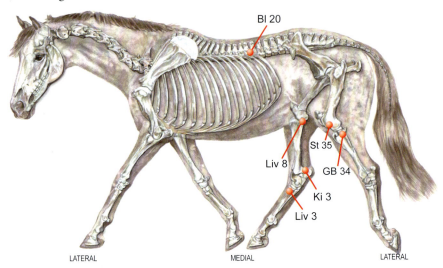

Point	Name	Location
St 35	Calf's Nose	In a depression between the middle and lateral patellar ligaments between the distal edge of the patella and the proximal edge of the tibia.
Bl 20	Spleen's Transport	Three cun lateral to the dorsal midline in the last (17th) intercostal space.
Ki 3	Great Stream	In the depression between the medial malleolus of the tibia and the tendocalcaneus. Opposite Bl 60.
Liv 3	Great Thoroughfare	On the craniodistal aspect of the cannon bone at the level of the head of the medial splint bone.
Liv 8	Crooked Spring	Behind the medial condyle of the femur, in front of the tendons of the semimembranosus and semitendinosus.
GB 34	Yang Mound Spring	In the interosseous space between the tibia and fibula between the long and lateral digital extensors, craniodistal to the head of the fibula.

TYING-UP
aka Azoturia, Myoglobinuria or Acute Exertional Rhabdomyolysis

This condition has earned many vernacular and technical names in just about every country over hundreds of years. No matter what it's called, tying-up is dangerous and painful for your equine athlete. It's usually associated with a horse exceeding his level of conditioning or experiencing intense exertion followed by confinement.

If you suspect your horse is in the process of tying-up, contact your veterinarian immediately – it is a serious condition and possibly life threatening.

The indicators of Tying-up can be as simple as a decrease in performance and as frightening as the horse passing dark red-brown colored urine, laying down in shock, or thrashing in pain. In mild and sporadic cases of Tying-up the horse usually exhibits some stiffness, shortened gait, possibly camping-out position and pain especially in hindquarter muscles. Unfortunately, even in mild cases there can be a breakdown in muscle cells causing muscle dysfunction and permanent damage.

Severe cases of Tying-up can be life threatening. A horse with a severe case can have dark red-brown urination, which can cause kidney and muscle damage while passing through the body.

The following acupressure routine can be used to prevent tying-up after exertion. If your horses is exhibiting signs of tying-up, contact your veterinarian and follow her recommendations before proceeding with this acupressure session.

Tying Up

Indicators

- Heightened heart and respiration rates
- Dehydration from excessive sweating
- Hard, stiff, painful muscles
- Inability to move
- Extreme thrashing in pain
- Shock

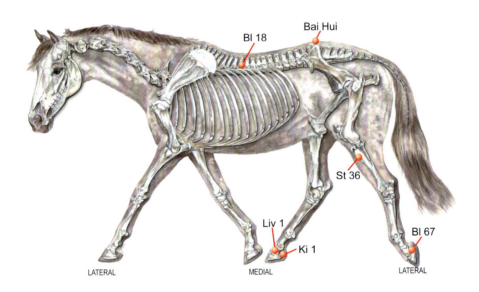

Point	Name	Location
St 36	Leg 3 Miles	One half (0.5) cun lateral to the tibial crest on the lateral side of the tibia.
Bl 18	Liver's Transport	Three cun lateral to the dorsal midline in the 13th and 14th intercostal spaces.
Bl 67	Reaching Yin	Found at the caudolateral aspect of the coronary band on the hind leg.
Ki 1	Gushing Spring	On the hind leg, in the depression between the heel bulbs.
Liv 1	Big Mound	On the craniomedial aspect of the hind hoof proximal to the coronary band.
Bai Hui	100 Meetings	On the dorsal midline at the lumbosacral space.

EQUINE REPRODUCTION

There are so many reasons for a mare to have fertility issues. It could be a hormonal imbalance, cysts, endometriosis to name a few. Have your holistic veterinarian or an equine reproduction specialist check your mare if she is experiencing a fertility or estrous cycle problem.

In Chinese medicine the Kidney governs reproduction and stores Source chi, which is the Original chi of the foal's body. It is the Essence chi the foal inherits from the dam and the sire that determines her eventual capacity to reproduce. It's important to support the health of the Liver and Conception Vessel because they play a significant role in fertility and reproduction as well.

The following acupressure session is intended to support the health and enhance the fertility of your broodmare.

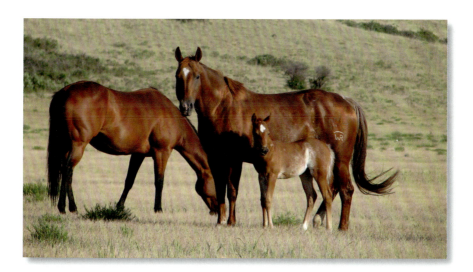

Fertility Issues

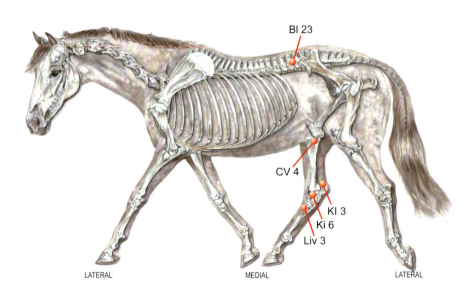

Point	Name	Location
Bl 23	Kidney's Transport	Three cun lateral to the dorsal midline between the 2nd and 3rd lumbar vertebrae directly dorsal to the ventral end of the last rib.
Ki 3	Great Stream	In the depression between the medial malleolus of the tibia and the calcaneal tuber. Opposite Bl 60.
Ki 6	Luminous Sea	In a depression between the calcaneal tuber and the talus.
Liv 3	Great Thoroughfare	On the craniodistal aspect of the cannon bone at the level of the head of the medial splint bone.
CV 4	Gate to Original Chi	On the ventral midline 3 cun caudal to the umbilicus.

INSUFFICIENT LACTATION

The mare's ability to nurse her foal is critical for the young life. The foal receives essential proteins and colostrum from his mother's milk. This is how the foal attains his initial antibodies to build his immune system. The balance of fat, protein, and lactose (sugar) in the mare's milk is perfect for the growth of the foal. The acupressure session below is suggested to support the health of the mare's mammary glands to ensure there's sufficient nutrient-rich milk for her foal.

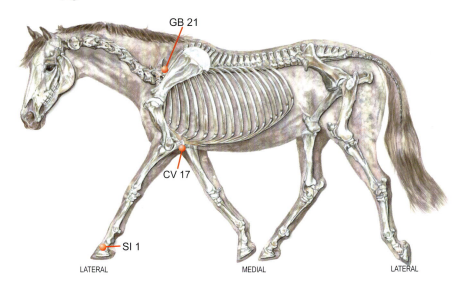

Point	Name	Location
SI 1	Young Marsh	On the craniolateral aspect of the front hoof proximal to the coronary band.
GB 21	Shoulder Well	At the midpoint of the cranial edge of the scapula.
CV 17	Sea of Tranquility	On the ventral midline at the level of the caudal border of the elbow.

ACU-HORSE: A GUIDE TO EQUINE ACUPRESSURE

RESPIRATORY CONDITIONS

The Lung is the most vulnerable of the organs to external pathogens. When airborne pathogens enter the body, Lung function can be compromised. The Lung plays an extremely important role in the strength of the immune system. Defensive chi, or *Wei chi,* is based on the proper functioning of the Lung. Keep in mind, no breath no life!

According to Chinese medicine, the Lung is responsible for descending chi. The Kidney must be strong enough to grasp the Lung chi and "root the breath." As horses age, the relationship between Lung and Kidney weakens. Older animals don't breathe as deeply; their breath can be shallow. This in turn affects stamina and strength. However, the relationship between Lung and Kidney sustains life until the very last exhale.

A general approach to respiratory issues is to maintain a strong immune system. (Refer to the Immune System Strengthening specific condition included in this chapter to ward off susceptibility to illness.) When your horse exhibits a respiratory issue, have your veterinarian examine him and follow any recommendations he or she gives. There are specific acupoints that directly support Lung function. The acupressure session below can be administered in conjunction with your veterinarian's recommendations.

General Indicators of Respiratory Conditions
- Sneezing
- Wheezing
- Hacking / Coughing
- Labored breathing
- Gurgling or rattling sound
- Gasping for breath
- Open mouth breathing
- Discharge from nose and/or eyes
- Choking up foam
- Blue lips, tongue, or gums
- Lethargy or weakness
- Fever
- Loss of appetite

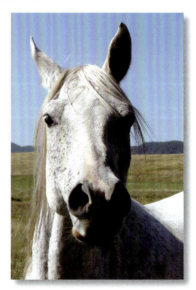

180

General Lung Support

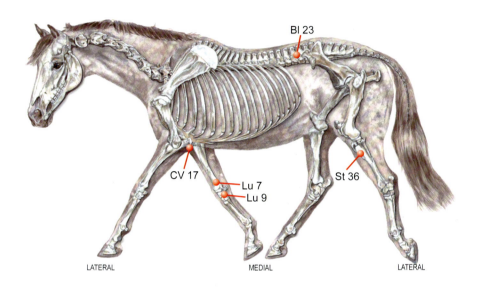

Point	Name	Location
Lu 7	Broken Sequence	Located just cranial to the cephalic vein at the level of the distal border of the chestnut.
Lu 9	Great Abyss	Located in the middle of the medial aspect of the foreleg, on the radial side of the carpus, between the 1st and 2nd row of carpal bones just cranial to the accessory carpal bone.
St 36	Leg 3 Miles	One half (0.5) cun lateral to the tibial crest on the lateral side of the tibia.
Bl 23	Kidney's Transport	Three cun lateral to the dorsal midline between the 2nd and 3rd lumbar vertebrae directly dorsal to the ventral end of the last rib.
CV 17	Sea of Tranquility	On the ventral midline at the level of the caudal border of the elbow.

Heaves
aka Recurrent Airway Obstruction (RAO)

Heaves is the most common respiratory disease in horses. It's most often seen in mature and older horses. Heaves is caused by an allergic reaction to an inhalant allergen such as dust or pollen. The cells in the lining of the horse's lungs swell and thicken due to inflammation in response to the allergen. As the disease progresses it becomes harder for the horse to breathe. Mucous forms in the air-passages causing coughing, bronchial muscle contraction, and nasal discharge. Because the horse has to work hard to exhale consistently the abdominal muscles become enlarged to form a characteristic "heaves line."

Unfortunately, there's no cure for heaves, but it's manageable. There are varying degrees of severity and the sooner the condition is recognized and treated the better. Horses can improve when they are no longer exposed to the irritant. Plus, offering an acupressure session to improve lung function by reducing inflammation, improving the flexibility of the air-passages, and removing the excess fluid can effectively eliminate the clinical signs of heaves. By combining this routine with the removal of the allergen from the horse's environment you can achieve a good level of recovery.

Indicators

- Cough
- Nasal discharge
- Labored, difficult breathing
- Congested breathing
- Wheezing sound on exhale
- Exercise intolerance
- Loss of weight
- Evidence of "heaves line"
- Low immune system

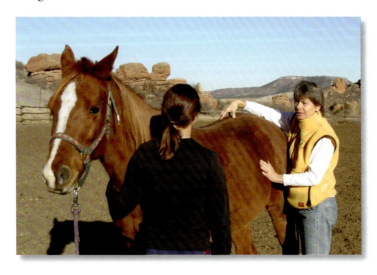

Heaves

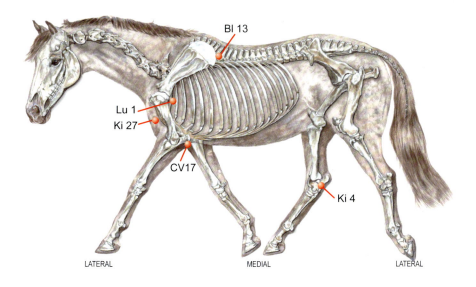

Point	Name	Location
Lu 1	Central Palace	Located in the depression in the center of the muscle belly of the descending pectoral muscle at the level of the 1st intercostal space.
Bl 13	Lung's Transport	Three cun lateral to the dorsal midline in the 8th intercostal space.
Ki 4	Big Bell	Found 0.5 cun caudodistal to Ki 3 on the medial border of the Achilles tendon.
Ki 27	Elegant Mansion	Located between the sternum and the 1st rib 2 cun lateral to the ventral midline.
CV 17	Sea of Tranquility	On the ventral midline at the level of the caudal border of the elbow.

SENSORY ISSUES
Visual Acuity

As a flight animal, horses rely on their eyes for cues. They have 65° of binocular vision and 285° of monocular vision. Their eyes are the largest of any mammal. The placement on the equine head allows for seeing a predator even while grazing. Any loss of visual acuity due to injury, illness, or degeneration can cause a horse to feel insecure, act-out, or reluctant to participate in activity. Untreated, even minor injuries or disease can result in blindness – have your veterinarian check any suspicious eye issue.

Indicators
- Not responsive to visual cues
- Shying unpredictably (hyper-reactive)
- Swelling
- Redness
- Squinting
- Abnormal discharge
- Reluctance to engage in activity

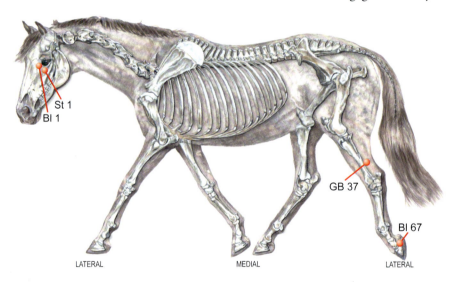

Point	Name	Location
St 1	Containing Tears	Directly below (ventral to) the center of the pupil.
Bl 1	Eye's Clarity	In the indentation at the medial canthus of the eye.
GB 37	Bright Light	Five cun above the tip of the lateral malleolus on the anterior border of the fibula.
Bl 67	Reaching Yin	Found at the caudolateral aspect of the coronary band on the hind leg.

Conjunctivitis

Indicators

- Swelling of the eye
- Yellow/white discharge from the eye
- Sticky eyelid
- Closed or squinting eye
- Pink or red mucous membrane (conjunctiva)
- Adverse response to bright light
- Adverse reaction to dust
- Rubbing eyes or shaking head

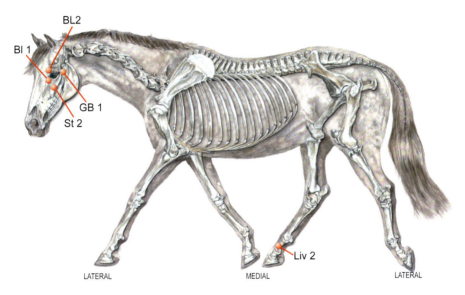

Point	Name	Location
St 2	Four Brightness	Located ventral to the medial canthus at the bifurcation of the angular vein.
Bl 1	Eye's Clarity	In the indentation at the medial canthus of the eye.
Bl 2	Collection of Bamboo	One cun dorsal to Bl 1 on the upper eyelid.
GB 1	Pupil's Seam	Located one cun caudoventral to the lateral canthus of the eye.
Liv 2	Travel Between	On the medial aspect of hind limb below the fetlock joint.

TRAUMA

Western conventional medicine is well equipped to handle traumatic events. Modern technology is essential in caring for your horse in a life-threatening situation. While waiting for veterinary care, if you can work with your horse safely, you can help mitigate the effects of the trauma using acupoints specific to the issue. These acupressure charts are a support, not a substitute, for veterinary trauma care.

All emergency events require immediate veterinary care!

ANHIDROSIS
aka Non-Sweating Disease

Anhidrosis is a serious syndrome which occurs when the horse's body heat builds up while exercising and sweat is not cooling the body. The internal heat can't escape and the horse's organs can fail and brain damage can occur. It can happen to any horse any time though it's more common in hot, humid, climates. Anhidrosis can occur suddenly or over a long period of time.

Acupressure has proven to be a good resource for helping horses exhibiting clinical signs of anhidrosis.

Indicators

- Patchy or no sweating after heavy exercise
- Elevated temperature, respiratory and/or pulse rate
- Slow recovery from a work-out
- Lethargic especially in a hot, humid climate
- Flaky skin and loss of coat
- Poor performance (reluctance to work)
- Loss of appetite
- Less water consumption than needed

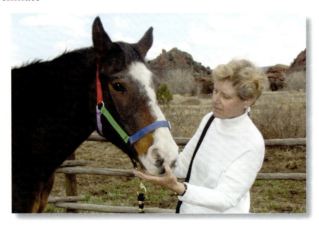

ANHIDROSIS

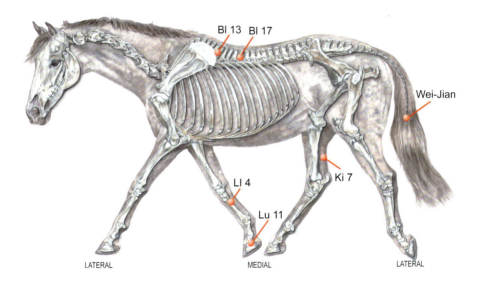

Point	Name	Location
Lu 11	Lesser Metal's Note	Located on the caudomedial aspect of the forelimb, proximal to the coronary band.
LI 4	Adjoining Valley	Found distal and medial to the head of the medial splint bone.
Bl 13	Lung's Transport	Three cun lateral to the dorsal midline in the 8th intercostal space.
Bl 17	Diaphragm's Transport	Three cun lateral to the dorsal midline in the 12th intercostal space.
Ki 7	Repeated Current	About 2 cun above Ki 3 on the cranial border of the Achilles tendon.
Wei Jian	Tip of Tail	At the tip of the tail, last caudal vertebra.

Heatstroke

When a horse is experiencing heatstroke – it's an extreme emergency. Your first action is to hose him down with running water (no ice) in the shade with a breeze or fans blowing to cool him down. Call your veterinarian and follow recommendations before offering the following acupressure routine. Heatstroke can result in your horse's internal organs shutting down – it's life-threatening.

Indicators

- Elevated body temperature
- Profuse sweating or hot dry coat
- Pale gums
- Dehydration
- Extreme lethargy, slow, stumbling
- Elevated heart rate
- Rapid breathing
- Diaphragm and/or flank muscle spasms
- Convulsions
- Collapse
- Unresponsiveness

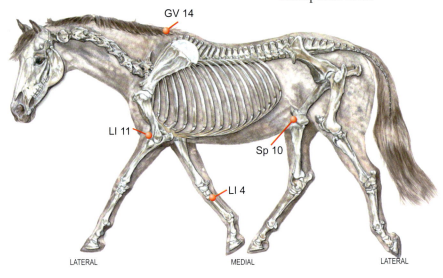

Point	Name	Location
LI 4	Adjoining Valley	Found distal and medial to the head of the medial splint bone.
LI 11	Crooked Pond	On the lateral aspect of the foreleg in a depression cranial to the elbow in the transverse cubital crease.
Sp 10	Sea of Blood	On the medial aspect of hind limb 2 cun proximal to the border of the patella, in the vastus medialis muscle.
GV 14	Big Vertebra	On the dorsal midline in a depression between the 7th cervical and 1st thoracic vertebrae cranial to the highest point of the withers.

Shock

Shock is an acute life-threatening condition where the horse's circulatory system is shutting down which deprives the body of oxygen leading to organ failure and death.

Seek veterinary care immediately! The acupoints given below are emergency points, but are not a substitute for immediate veterinary attention.

Indicators

- Rapid or shallow breathing
- Major physical injury
- Severe colic
- Extreme pain
- Shaking or shivering
- Weak pulse
- Blood loss
- Poor capillary refill (more than 2 seconds)
- Cold extremities and ears
- Loss of consciousness

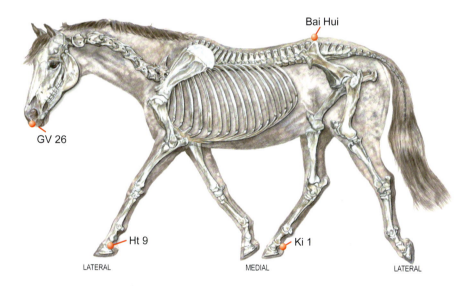

Point	Name	Location
Ht 9	Lesser Rushing	On the caudolateral aspect of the front hoof proximal to the coronary band.
Ki 1	Gushing Spring	On the hind leg in depression between the heel bulbs.
Bai Hui	100 Meetings	On the dorsal midline at the lumbosacral space.
GV 26	Middle of Man	On dorsal midline between ventral limits of the nostrils.

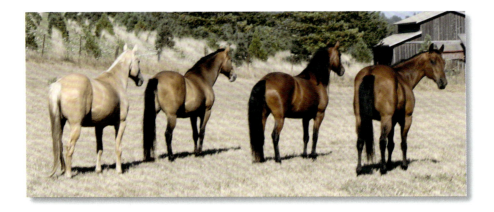

There is something about the outside of a horse that is good for the inside of a man.
— Winston Churchill

Glossary

Abdominal cavity The cavity of the body located between the diaphragm and the pelvis. This cavity contains the abdominal organs.

Acetabulum The socket portion of the ball-and-socket hip joint. It is formed at the junction of the ilium, ischium and pubis bones of the pelvis. The cup-shaped socket of the hip joint that carries the head of the femur.

Acupoint Specific acupoints located on a meridian where chi flows close to the surface of the body. Stimulation, tonification, sedation and other techniques can be employed to manipulate the chi energy of the body at these locations. There are 361 acupoints located along the 12 Major Meridians.

Acupressure An ancient healing art that moves and balances chi and blood by use of pressure applied at specific acupoints along the meridian system. Used to release muscular pain, tension, to increase circulation and treat a variety of ailments and conditions by balancing vital substances.

Acupuncture The manipulation of chi energy by use of needle insertions at specific acupoints along the meridian system. Used to release muscular pain, tension, to increase circulation and treat a variety of ailments and conditions by balancing vital substances.

Acute A condition having a short and relatively sudden course, not long-term.

Alarm point A classification of acupoints where the chi energy of a particular organ accumulates when the organ is imbalanced. Alarm points are used in both assessment and treatment and are often used in conjunction with the Association points.

Glossary

Annular ligament A ligament that wraps around a structure.

Anti-inflammatory An agent that relieves inflammation or swelling, and heat, of the tissues.

Artery The blood vessel carrying blood away from the heart into the system. The blood vessels furnish oxygen and nutrients to the body tissues.

Articulate To join or unite by joints.

Association point A classification of points located along the inner channel of the Bladder meridian. Each of the 12 Major Meridians has a unique Association point that exhibits an internal / external relationship with each of the organs. These points can indicate a blockage in their corresponding meridian and are often used in conjunction with the Alarm points to help identify the level of organ involvement.

Atlas The first cervical vertebra (C 1). It forms the atlanto-occipital joint with the occipital bone of the skull and the atlantoaxial joint with the axis C 2).

Atrophy Decrease in size of muscle or organ resulting from lack of use or disease.

Autoimmune disease Refers to a variety of serious, chronic illnesses where the body's immune system becomes misdirected, attacking the organs it was designed to protect.

Axis The second cervical vertebra (C 2). It is the longest of the vertebrae in the column.

Axilla The armpit.

Glossary

Belly — The thick, central portion of a muscle.

Blood — In TCM, the red liquid which circulates in the vessels, and is a vital nutrient substance in the body, *Xue*.

Body fluid — In TCM, the collective term for all the normal fluids of the body. These include saliva, gastric juice, intestinal juice, and the liquids of the joint cavities, as well as tears, nasal discharge, sweat, and urine.

Calcaneus — The irregular quadrangular bone located at the back of the hock, part of which points upward and backward to form the point of the hock.

Cannon — The area between the knee or hock, and the knee and fetlock. The canon bone is the 3rd metacarpal / metatarsal of the horse.

Capsular ligament — The fibrous layer of a joint capsule.

Cartilage — A dense, gristly, type of connective tissue found on the articular ends of bones.

Carpus — The segment of limb between the radius and the ulna and the metacarpus, made up of 7 - 8 bones. These bones are arranged in two rows known as the knee in horses.

Caudal — Situated more toward the tail than some specific reference point.

Caudal vertebrae — The 5th region of the vertebral column consisting of 18 - 26 vertebrae, forming the tail. Also known as coccygeal vertebrae.

Glossary

Central nervous system	The brain and spinal cord.
Cervical vertebrae	The seven bones of the neck portion of the spinal column, includes the atlas and the axis.
Channel chi	The aspect of chi that flows through the meridian or channel system. It is the aspect of chi that is most available for adjustment or influence by acupressure or acupuncture.
Chi	Life-promoting energy present in all of nature. There are different types of chi, defined by location and function.
Chronic	A condition that persists for a long time with little change or improvement.
Closing	The third phase of an acupressure session. The closing serves to connect the energy flow between the acupoints stimulated during the session. It also repatterns cellular memory and benefits chronic pain.
Coccygeal vertebrae	The 5th region of the vertebral column located at the tail, also known as the caudal vertebrae.
Condyle	A rounded projection on a bone, mostly for articulation with another bone.
Conception Vessel	One of the eight Extraordinary Vessels. A yin vessel running along the ventral midline.
Connecting point	A classifications of acupoints that connect the Yin and Yang energies of the sister meridians. These points help resolve blockages between the sister meridians and enhance point work.

Glossary

Conjunctivitis — Inflammation of the mucous membrane that lines the exposed portion of the eyeball and inner surface of the eyelids.

Connective tissue — A fibrous type of body tissue. This tissue supports and connects the internal organs, forms bones and the walls of blood vessels. It also attaches muscles to bones, and replaces other types of tissue after injury.

Control Cycle — The sequence of the Five-Element Theory in which each element controls another and is itself controlled by another element. This sequence helps ensure balance is maintained among the five elements. Also called the *Ko* cycle.

Coronary band — The junction of the skin and the horn of the hoof. It encircles the hoof.

Costal arch — The rim to the bony thorax formed by the conjoined asternal ribs and their connecting elastic tissue.

Cranial — The position of a point or structure toward the head, the front or superior end of the body.

Creation Cycle — The sequence of the Five-Element Theory in which each element creates another and is itself created by another element. This sequence helps ensure that a balance is maintained among the five elements. Also called *Sheng* cycle.

Cun — Translates to 'little measurement'. Used to help define a more exact location for acupressure points on the body.

Cutaneous — Pertaining to the skin.

Glossary

Deficiency — A condition of insufficiency or too little of a vital substance.

Distal — Refers to structures or points that lie furthest away from the body or trunk. Opposite of proximal.

Distal point — Acupressure points located away from the area they benefit. For instance, Liv 2 is a distal point when used to strengthen the eyes.

Dorsal — An area directed toward or situated on the back surface, the surface facing away from the ground.

Dysuria — Painful or difficult urination.

Endocrine system — The system of glands that controls and regulates body functions through the internal secretion of hormones, which are placed directly into the bloodstream where they act throughout the body.

Essence — Also called *Jing*, housed in the Kidney, the substance of the body.

Estrous — The entire reproductive cycle of the animal. Regularly occurring periods during which the mare is sexually active and receptive. Anestrous is the lack of estrous.

Excess — A condition of surplus or too much of something, such as chi, blood, body fluids, etc.

Extension — The joint movement that increase the angle between two bones.

Extensor muscles — Any muscle that extends a joint.

External — This term refers to all that is outside the body. Located on or near the outside.

Glossary

Extraordinary Vessels — Eight vessels which act as reservoirs of energy for the major meridians. They absorb energy from the major meridians or transfer energy to the major meridians as needed.

Femorotibial joint — The joint of the femur and tibia.

Femur — The thigh bone, which runs from the pelvis to the stifle.

Flexion — The act of bending or the condition of being bent.

Flexor muscle — Any muscle that flexes a joint.

Fibula — The smaller and lateral of the two bones of the lower end of the hind limb, from stifle to hock. Does not support any appreciable weight, mainly a muscle attachment site.

Five Phases of Transformation — A conceptual framework representative of the natural phases of transformation and cycles of life and seasonal/environmental changes.

Foramen — A hole in a bone.

Fossa — A hollow or depressed area, a trench or groove like channel.

Fu organs — The six Yang organs, also referred to as the hollow organs: Large Intestine, Stomach, Small Intestine, Bladder, Triple Heater, and Gall Bladder.

Gait — The manner or style of locomotion. Used often to assess the soundness of an animal. Gaits include the walk, trot, amble, pace, canter, and gallop.

Glossary

Gastrointestinal	Pertaining to the stomach and intestines, it can refer to the entire digestive tract.
Hindquarters	The body area located behind the flanks and includes the pelvis, thighs, hocks and the muscular area of the hind legs.
Head	A spheroidal articular surface on the proximal end of a long bone. A head is present on the proximal ends of the humerus, femur and rib. The head of a bone is joined to the shaft by an area that is often narrowed, called the neck.
Hock joint	The tarsal joint. The area of the tarsus on the hind limb of the horse, corresponding to the ankle joint of humans.
Humero radial	Pertaining to the humerus and radius, two bones of the thoracic limb.
Influential point	A classification of acupoints which affect a particular functional system of the body.
Ilium	The largest of the three bones of the pelvis.
Intercostal	Between the ribs.
Intervertebral	Between two vertebrae.
Intervertebral disk	The cartilaginous disk located between the bodies of adjacent vertebrae. Acts as a shock absorber for the vertebrae.
Jing	The life essence, or material aspect of chi, a fundamental substance stored in the kidney.

Glossary

Jing-Well point A classification of acupoints located at the coronary band of the horse's front and hind legs. There is one Jing-Well point for each meridian. Used to balance the meridian and for other specific conditions.

Joint The union or junction of two or more bones. Main function of a joint is to provide motion, flexibility, absorb concussion and allow for growth. Joints can be completely immovable, slightly movable (cartilaginous joints), or freely movable (synovial joints).

Jugular groove The groove or furrow on each side of the neck in which the jugular vein is located, dorsal to the trachea.

Lame An irregularity or impairment of the function of locomotion or gait.

Laminae Layers of fibrous tissue on the inside of the hoof wall.

Lateral Anatomical term for points or structures that are situated further away from the midline or median plane of the body.

Ligament A band of fibrous tissue that connects bone or cartilages or supports viscera and serves to support and strengthen joints.

Local point Acupressure points located in the area they benefit. For example, GB 1 and Bl 1 are local points for the eye.

Lumbar Pertaining to the loins, the part of the back between the thorax and pelvis.

Lumbosacral joint The junction between the last lumbar vertebrae and the sacrum.

Glossary

Lung chi	Life energy, chi is extracted from the air and transformed to bioavailable chi in the Lung.
Lymphatic system	The system that collects lymph from the tissues and returns it to the general circulation.
Mandible	The bone that forms the lower jaw.
Manubrium	The most cranial portion of the sternum.
Marrow	In TCM, a substance which is the common matrix of bones, bone marrow, the brain, and the spinal cord. The Kidney-Essence produces Marrow which generates the spinal cord and "fills up" the brain. The Marrow is also the basis for the formation of bone marrow which nourishes the bones. The Kidneys also govern the bone marrow and bones.
Master point	A classification of acupoints which affect a regional area of the body. There are 6 Master points.
Maxilla	One of two identical bones that forms the upper jaw. These bones meet at the facial midline, often considered one bone.
Medial	Points or structures that are situated nearer to the midline or median plane of the body.
Meridian blockage	A condition which impedes the smooth, even, and balanced flow of chi throughout the meridian system.
Meridian system	The network of invisible but real channels through which the chi flows throughout the body. These channels are located just below the skin and are connected and influence each other.

Glossary

Meridians Individual energy pathways, or channels, that are part of a body wide network through which chi and blood flow.

Metacarpal bones The bones comprised of the front cannon and splint bones, the 3rd metacarpal bone (cannon is a strong and long weight-bearing bone. The 2nd and 4th metacarpal bones are thin, non weight-bearing vestigial bones.

Muscle An organ made up of bundles of fiber that have the power to contract and therefore to produce movement. Muscles function to provide locomotion and support for the body. There are voluntary and involuntary muscles.

Myositis Inflammation of a voluntary muscle. Causes heat, swelling pain, and lameness if a limb is affected.

Navicular syndrome Degenerative condition of the navicular bone and/or its supporting structures.

Nephritis Inflammation of the Kidney.

Nutrient chi Also known as *Ying* or *Gu chi*. It is the chi obtained from food.

Nuchal ligament The powerful elastic apparatus that serves to support the head without muscular effort. It joins the axis to the withers and is continuous with the thorocolumbar part of the supraspinous ligament

Opening The first phase of an acupressure session. The Opening introduces 'structured' touch, provides feedback to the practitioner, is used for assessment and session work.

Glossary

Origin — The more fixed end or attachment of a muscle or the end closer to the trunk. This provides stability so that the insertion of the muscle can move bones or other structures.

Original chi — The more fixed end or attachment of a muscle or the end closer to the trunk. This provides stability so that the insertion of the muscle can move bones or other structures.

Palpation — To examine or explore by touching usually as an assessment tool.

Patella — The kneecap. A large sesamoid bone at the femorotibial joint.

Pectoral — Pertaining to the chest or breast area.

Pelvic limb — Either hind leg.

Pelvis — The bony girdle comprised of the ilium, ischium, and pubis.

Point of hock — The summit of the calcaneus. The calcaneon tuber.

Point Work — The 2nd phase of an acupressure session, when acupoints located along the meridian system are stimulated.

Point Work Techniques — The procedures used to stimulate points. There are several techniques a practitioner may use each has a unique stimulating quality.

Protective chi — The chi that protects the body from harmful external forces or pathogens.

Glossary

Proximal Refers to structures or points that lie nearest to the body or trunk.

Rostral Structures or points that are located closer to the nose. Generally used to describe positions and directions only on the head.

Sacral vertebrae The vertebrae of the pelvic region. The are fused into a solid structure called the sacrum. The sacrum forms a joint with the ilium of the pelvis on each side called the sacroiliac joint.

Sacroiliac joint The joint between the pelvis and the sacrum that joins the pelvic limb to the axial skeleton.

Sacrum The 4th segment of the bertebral column, made up of five fused sacral vertebrae.

Scapula The flat triangular shaped bone comprising the shoulder. In domestic animals, no bony connection exists between the scapula and the axial skeleton.

Scapulo humeral joint The articular surface between the scapula and the humerus.

Sedate To disperse or decrease.

Sesamoid bone A bone present in some tendons where they change direction markedly over joints. They act as bearings over the joint surfaces, allowing powerful muscles to move the joints without the tendons wearing out as they move over the joints.

Shen Represents the 'spirit' or consciousness aspect of the animal.

Glossary

Shock — A condition of acute peripheral circulatory failure due to derangement of circulatory control or loss of circulating fluid.

Six Exogenous Pathogenic Factors — Exogenous pathogenic factors can invade the body and cause disease when chi is weak or sudden change in climate and the horse's body cannot adapt and they include: Wind, Cold, Wet Dry, Hot/Fire, and Summer Heat.

Skeleton — The bony framework of the body. There are typically about 205 bones in the skeleton of a horse.

Skeletal muscle — Striated, voluntary muscle that enables conscious movement. The type of muscle that moves the bones of the skeleton.

Smooth muscle — Nonstriated, involuntary muscle having only one nucleus. The type of muscle found in soft internal organs and structures. Not under conscious control.

Source point — A classification of points that either sedate or tonify, depending upon the need of the meridian at the time of stimulation. There is a Source point for each meridian and it is where Original, or Source chi, can be accessed.

Spinous processes — The upward projections of each vertebrae.

Sternal ribs — Ribs that are attached to the sternum.

Sternum — A longitudinal, unpaired plate of bone forming the middle of the ventral wall of the thorax. It has three parts, the manubrium, the body and the xiphoid process.

Glossary

Stifle — The 'knee' on the hind leg of the horse. Formed by the lower end of the tibia with the kneecap (patella) attached to the front.

Striated muscle — Mainly attached to the skeleton. Their movements are under the conscious control of the individual, and are involved with such things as walking, eating, tail swishing, eye movement, etc.

Superficial — Structures that occur near the surface of the body.

Suspensory ligament — A ligament whose function is to support or hold up a part of the body or an organ.

Synovial fluid — The yellow-white transparent viscous fluid secreted by the synovial membrane and found in joint cavities, bursae and tendon sheaths. It serves to lubricate moving parts and nourish articular cartilage.

Tarsus — The joint of the distal hind limb. It is composed of numerous, small short bones. The proximal border of the tarsus articulates with the tibia and fibula.

Tendon — A fibrous cord which attaches muscles to bones or other structure. When the muscle contracts, the tendon is pulled. Serve to convey an action to a remote site, change the direction of pull, and focus the energy.

Tetany — Continuous tonic spasm of a muscle; steady contraction of a muscle without distinct twitching. Manifested by rigidity of limbs, pricking of ears or flaring of nostrils.

Thoracic cavity — The chest cavity. It is separated from the abdominal cavity by the thin, sheet like diaphragm.

Glossary

Thoracic limb	The front limb.
Thoracic vertebrae	The 2nd segment of the vertebral column, made up of 18 vertebrae. Located between the cervical and lumbar vertebrae.
Thorax	The part of the body between the neck and the abdomen. The chest. Separated from the abdomen by the diaphragm, walls are formed by pairs of ribs.
Tibia	The larger and inner bone of the hind limb, below the stifle. The main weight bearing bone of the lower leg.
Tibial crest	A longitudinal ridge on the front of the proximal end of the tibia.
TMJ	Temporomandibular joint, the hinge joint on each side of the lower jaw that connects it with the rest of the skull.
Tonify	To increase or strengthen.
Trochanter	One of the three tuberosities on the femur. The greater trochanter is located at its upper end on the lateral surface, the lesser trochanter is located toward the upper end on its medial surface and the third trochanter is located distally on the lateral surface.
Tuber coxae	The point of the hip, the most lateral point of the ilium. Also called the coxal tuber.
Tuber sacrale	The most prominent medial prominence on the ilium, above the sacroiliac joint.

Glossary

Tuberosity — An elevation or protuberance on a bone to which muscles are attached.

Ulna — Smaller of two bones of forearm, upper part of which forms the point of the elbow (olecranon).

Ventral — Directed toward or situated on the belly surface toward the ground. The opposite of dorsal.

Vertebra — Any of the separate segments comprising the spine. They support the body and provide the protective bony corridor through which the spinal cord passes.

Vital Substance — Substances processed and stored in the Yin organs. These substances include chi, shen, essence, blood, and body fluids.

Xiphoid process — The pointed process of cartilage connected with the posterior end of the body of the sternum.

Zang Organs — The six yin organs, also referred to at the solid organs: Lung, Spleen, Heart, Kidney Pericardium, and Liver.

Zygomatic arch — The bony arch below and behind the eyes of common domestic animals, formed by the processos of the zygomatic and temporal bones.

Bibliography

Altman, Sheldon, DVM. *An Introduction to Acupuncture for Animals.* Chen's Corporation, Monterey Park, CA. 1981.

Beinfield, Harriet, L.Ac. & Korngold, Efrem, L. Ac., OMD. *Between Heaven and Earth, A Guide to Chinese Medicine.* Ballentine Books, New York, NY. 1991.

Birch, Stephen and Matsumoto, Kiiko, *Five Elements and Ten Stems.* Paradigm Publications, Brookline, MA. 1983.

Budiansky, Stephen, *The Nature of Horses.* The Free Press/Simon & Schuster Inc., New York, 1997.

Cohen, Misha Ruth, OMD, Lac. *The Chinese Way to Healing: Many Paths to Wholeness.* A Perigree Book, The Berkley Publishing Group, New York, NY. 1996.

International Veterinary Acupuncture Society, *The Chinese Acupuncture, 5,000 Year Old Oriental Art of Healing.*

Kaselle, Marion and Hannay, Pamela, *Touching Horses.* J.A.Allen & Co Ltd, London, 1995.

Maoshing Ni, Ph.D. *The Yellow Emperor's Classic of Medicine;* New Translation of the Neijing Suwen with Commentary. Shambhala Publications, Inc. Boston, MA. 1995.

Maciocia, Giovanni, CaC. *The Foundations of Chinese Medicine, A Comprehensive Text for Acupuncturists and Herbalist, Second Editions.* Churchill Livingstone (Elsevier Limited), 2005.

Mann, Felix, MB. *Acupuncture, The Ancient Chinese Art of Healing and How It Works Scientifically.* Vintage Books, New York, NY. 1973.

Schoen,Allen,M. *Veterinary Acupuncture, Ancient Art to Modern Medicine, Second Edition. Mosby (Elsevier affiliate).St. Louis, MO. 2001.*

Schoen, Allen M., DVM, MS and Wynn, Susan, DVM. *Complimentary and Alternative Veterinary Medicine.*Mosby (*Elsevier affiliate).* 1998.

Snow, Amy and Zidonis, Nancy, *Acu-Cat: A Guide to Feline Acupressure.* Tallgrass Publishers, LLC., Colorado, 2012

Snow, Amy and Zidonis, Nancy, *Acu-Dog: A Guide to Canine Acupressure.* Tallgrass Publishers, LLC., Colorado, 2011.

Wiseman, Nigel, Ellis, Andrew. *Fundamentals of Chinese Medicine,* Revised Edition. Paradigm Publications, Brookline, Ma.1996.

Xie, Hulsheng,CVM, ph.D., MS, Preast, DVM, Vanessa. *Traditional Chinese Veterinary Medicine, Volume 1: Fundamental Principles.* Jing Tang. 2005.

Xie, Hulsheng,CVM, ph.D., MS, Preast, DVM, Vanessa. Xie's *Veterinary Acupuncture.* Blackwell Publishing. Ames, Iowa. 2007

Xinnong, Cheng. *Chinese Acupuncture and Moxibustion.* Foreign Language Press, Beijing, China. 1987

Yanchi, Liu. *The Essential Book of Traditional Chinese Medicine, Volume 1 Theory.* Columbia University Press, New York. 1988.

Index

A

acupressure protocol 118, 121
acupressure session 117, 118, 121, 130, 137
aging 32, 143, 144
Alarm point 108, 111, 112
allergies 18, 55, 58 63
alleviates pain 59, 60, 71, 77, 80, 85, 86
Anhidrosis 186
anxiety 61, 63, 64, 67, 68, 69, 70, 72, 73, 75, 78, 80, 81, 83, 84, 94, 96, 97, 151, 153, 156
arthritis 57, 65, 66, 69, 71, 77, 78, 80, 85, 89, 143, 145
Association point 108, 111
atrophy 31, 63, 74, 75, 76, 77, 86, 89

B

Barefoot Doctor 11
behavior 55, 58, 61, 64, 70, 90, 96, 150 152, 156
Bi Syndromes 167
blood deficiency 64, 116

C

cervical 74, 77, 86, 88, 99, 168
closing 137
colic 61, 63, 64, 65, 76, 85, 95, 98, 152, 158, 159, 160
compulsive behaviors 55, 58, 156
conception vessel 56, 93, 94, 96, 115
conjunctivitis 60, 74, 85, 96, 141, 185
constipation 58, 59, 62, 63, 66, 76, 79, 80, 91, 98, 162
cribbing 151, 152
cun measurement 12

D

Defensive chi 43, 55, 163, 180
deficiency 30, 31, 32, 57, 66, 68, 80, 81, 98, 99, a, 116, 145
deficiency 50
dental 58, 59, 60, 62, 63, 78, 86
diarrhea 21, 28, 58, 59, 60, 62, 63, 65, 66, 76, 79, 95, 98, 162
digestion 18, 30, 36, 70, 87, 90, 115, 158, 161
distal acupoints 141
dysuria 80, 95

E

Earth Element 36, 41, 105
edema 56, 60, 62, 64, 66, 76, 77, 80, 84, 85, 96, 149, 165
elbow pain 56
Emotional issues 58, 61, 64, 67, 70, 73, 78, 81, 84, 87, 90, 94
Essence 18, 44, 76, 78, 80, 93, 95 130 143, 177

Index

estrous 66, 76, 78, 80, 90, 91, 95, 177
excess 27, 28, 29, 50, 104, 105, 128, 129, 130, 182

F

fear 37, 73, 78, 96, 153
Fire Element 36, 67, 70, 81, 84
Five-Element Theory 33, 50
Focus for Training 154
Four Examinations 50, 102, 120, 132

G

Gall Bladder 87
gastrointestinal 62, 75, 76, 96, 161, 162
Governing Vessel 49, 93, 97
grief 37, 43, 55, 56, 58, 155

H

Heart 67
Heart chi 22, 67, 68
Heatstroke 79, 82, 83, 99, 188
Heaves 66, 80, 182
Herd behavior 5, 151
Hock issues 77, 169
hock problems 87
Hoof problems 59, 87

I

Immune system 84, 99, 103, 116, 129, 163, 164, 179, 180
Improve digestion 161
infection 21, 66, 105, 143, 164
Insufficient lactation 71, 82, 96, 179
internal pathogens 81
itchy skin 74

J

Jing 18, 78 143
Jing-Well point 57, 59, 63, 65, 69, 71, 77, 79, 83, 85, 91, 100

K

Kidney chi 78, 98, 123, 163
Kidney meridian 79

L

lameness 59, 60, 68, 69, 72, 77, 98, 101, 143, 145, 147, 166, 168, 169, 173, 174
Large Intestine meridian 58
Law of Integrity 14, 15, 16
Liver chi 75, 88, 89, 91, 92
Liver meridian 46, 47, 49, 91 130
local points 52, 141

Index

loss of consciousness 21, 69, 189
lower back soreness 73, 170
Lung meridian 51, 55, 111, 129, 139
Lung support 181

M

Master point 56, 59, 63, 66, 77, 82
Metal Element 37, 41, 55, 58
Musculoskeletal 101, 114, 141, 143, 167

N

neck pain 70, 71
nervousness 156
Nutrient chi 19, 20, 21, 48, 64

O

Opening 120, 121, 123, 124, 129, 137
organ prolapse 64, 95
Original chi 19, 84, 93, 94, 130, 177

P

Pattern of disharmony 22, 27, 28, 29, 32, 41, 42, 46, 50, 52, 102, 103, 105, 121, 124, 129, 139, 145

Pectoral chi 19, 20
Pericardium meridian 45, 81
Point Work 73, 130, 133, 134, 139
Point Work Technique 133, 135, 136
Post-Performance 172
Pre-Performance 171

R

reproduction 5, 15, 19, 78, 94, 177
Reproductive issues 90
Respiratory issues 9, 21, 52, 53, 180

S

seizures 21, 60, 63, 68, 69, 71, 72, 75, 76, 79, 80, 82, 87, 88, 90, 95, 96, 98, 99
Sensory orifice 36, 43, 55, 64, 67, 71, 74, 78, 85, 90
Shen 44, 67, 70, 78, 103, 143
Shen disturbance 67, 68, 69, 83, 99
Shock 63, 65, 83, 95, 99, 175, 176, 189
Shoulder soreness 173
Six Exogenous 21
Small Intestine meridian 70
Source chi 18, 19, 20, 80, 95, 98, 130, 177
Source point 57, 63, 65, 69, 71, 77, 83, 84, 85, 89, 91, 113, 130, 132, 139

Index

Spleen chi 115
Spleen meridian 64, 65
Stifle issues 61, 64, 78, 174
Stomach chi 22, 61
Stomach meridian 61, 62

T

tendinitis 71, 75, 89
tendon issues 72, 115
Theory of Chi 17, 32
Thumb Technique 134
TMJ 61, 64, 70, 86
toxins 163, 165, 172
Trauma 52, 53, 102, 143, 163, 186
Triple Heater meridian 85
True chi 19, 64
Two-finger Technique 134, 135
Tying Up 176

U

Universal Law 8, 13, 14, 16
urinary tract 66, 73, 78, 88

V

Visual acuity 47, 184
Vital substances 17, 26, 44, 47, 53

W

Water Element 37, 73, 78
Wei chi 17, 19, 20, 21, 61, 163, 180
Wood Element 35, 42, 87, 90

Y

Ying chi 19, 93
Yin-yang Theory 23, 42, 50, 103

Z

Zang-fu Theory 44, 46
Zheng chi 17, 20
Zong chi 19, 37, 43

Photographic Credits

Thank you to all the fine photographers who happily contributed the following photos of their favorite horses. We appreciate and enjoy including them in *ACU-HORSE*. If we have inadvertently missed crediting your photo, our apologies, and please let us know so we can update the list.

– Thank you!

Page	Photographer
Front Cover Photograph	John Wiet Photography
4, 5, 6, 15, 22, 116, 150, 167, 190	Barbara Chasteen
19	Gillian Magnabosco
52, 69, 83, 86, 109	Grant Dunmire
107, 163	Kim Bauer
151	Mike Brunfelt
103, 113, 120, 127	Grant Dunmire
Back Cover Photograph	John Wiet Photography

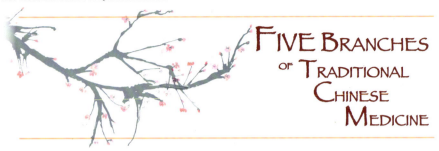

Five Branches of Traditional Chinese Medicine

From the perspective of this ancient medicine, everything is "medicine." Health is defined as both an internal and external balance of nutrients and energy so that the human and horse alike can function optimally within its environment. The intention is to support the body's capacity to adapt to constant change.

To achieve health and wellbeing, Chinese medicine incorporates five branches, or stems, as a guide to living a balanced life. Diet is essential. Exercise and body movement to enliven energy is absolutely necessary. All mammals need touch for sensory and caring stimulation. When imbalance threatens, further medicinal herbs and acupuncture and/or acupressure are necessary to restore the harmonious flow of chi and blood.

Five Branches of Traditional Chinese Medicine needed for a long, healthy life are:

- Diet
- Chi Gong – Exercise
- Tui Na – Chinese Meridian Acupressure-Massage
- Acupuncture
- Herbs

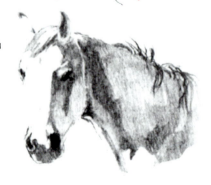

Author Profiles

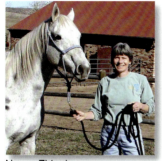
Nancy Zidonis

Nancy Zidonis and **Amy Snow** are the co-founders of Tallgrass Animal Acupressure Institute. The Institute offers hands-on and online certificate training programs worldwide. Nancy and Amy have authored feline, canine, and equine articles for numerous publications, books, and manuals including:

ACU-CAT: A Guide to Feline Acupressure, 2nd Ed.
ACU-DOG: A Guide to Canine Acupressure
Canine Acupoint Energetics & Landmark Anatomy
Canine Health & Pathology Manual
Equine Acupoint Energetics & Landmark Anatomy
Equine Acupressure: A Working Manual (out of print)
Equine Health & Pathology Manual
The Well-Connected Dog: A Guide to Canine Acupressure (out of print)

Additionally, they have produced four DVDs and meridian charts for horses, dogs, and cats. Most recently, they have produced apps for mobile devices – Equine AcuPoints and Canine AcuPoints. The apps are available through the Apple App Store and Google Play.

Both Nancy and Amy studied and practiced Traditional Chinese Medicine and have worked with animals for over 25 years. Their work reflects their intention of bringing animal acupressure to the people who can benefit animals most.

For more information:
www.animalacupressure.com

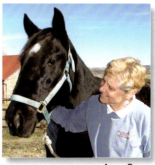
Amy Snow